HAND REHABILITATION

CLINICS IN PHYSICAL THERAPY
VOLUME 9

Already Published

Vol. 1 Cardiac Rehabilitation
Louis R. Amundsen, Ph.D., guest editor

Vol. 2 Electrotherapy
Steven L. Wolf, Ph.D., guest editor

Vol. 3 Physical Therapy of the Geriatric Patient
Osa Jackson, Ph.D., guest editor

Vol. 4 Rehabilitation of the Burn Patient
Vincent R. DiGregorio, M.D., guest editor

Vol. 5 Pediatric Neurologic Physical Therapy
Suzann K. Campbell, Ph.D., guest editor

Vol. 6 Spinal Cord Injury
Hazel V. Adkins, R.P.T., guest editor

Vol. 7 Measurement in Physical Therapy
Jules M. Rothstein, Ph.D., guest editor

Vol. 8 Psychosocial Aspects of Clinical Practice
Otto D. Payton, Ph.D., guest editor

Forthcoming Volumes in the Series

Vol. 10 Sports Physical Therapy
Donna Bernhardt, M.S., R.P.T., A.T.C., guest editor

Vol. 11   Pain
          John L. Echternach, Ed.D., guest editor

Vol. 12   Physical Therapy of the Knee
          Robert E. Mangine, M.Ed., L.P.T., guest editor

Vol. 13   Therapeutic Considerations for the Elderly
          Osa Jackson-Klykken, Ph.D., guest editor

Vol. 14   Physical Therapy for the Arthritis Patient
          Barbara Banwell, R.P.T., guest editor

Vol. 15   Physical Therapy of the Shoulder
          Robert Donatelli, M.A., R.P.T., guest editor

Vol. 16   Physical Therapy of the Foot and Ankle
          Gary C. Hunt, R.P.T., M.A., guest editor

Vol. 17   Craniomandibular Complex: Physical Therapy
          and Dental Management
          Steven L. Kraus, R.P.T., guest editor

Vol. 18   Physical Therapy of the Low Back
          Lance T. Twomey, B.App. Sc., B.Sc. (Hon),
          Ph.D., M.A.P.A., M.M.T.A.A., and James
          Taylor, M.B.Ch.B., Dip.Trop.Med., Ph.D.,
          guest editors

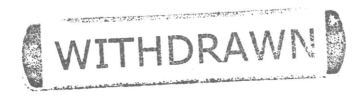

HAND REHABILITATION

Edited by

Christine A. Moran, M.S., R.P.T.

Director, The Richmond Upper Extremity Center
Assistant Clinical Professor of Physical Therapy
Medical College of Virginia
Virginia Commonwealth University
Richmond, Virginia

Adjunct Assistant Clinical Professor of
 Physical Therapy
Old Dominion University
Norfolk, Virginia

CHURCHILL LIVINGSTONE
NEW YORK, EDINBURGH, LONDON, MELBOURNE   1986

Acquisitions editor: Kim Loretucci
Copy editor: Michael Kelley
Production designer: Michiko Davis
Production supervisor: Joe Sita
Compositor: Eastern Graphics
Printer/Binder: The Maple-Vail Book Manufacturing Group

© Churchill Livingstone Inc. 1986

Distributed in the United Kingdom by Churchill Livingstone, Robert
Stevenson House, 1–3 Baxter's Place, Leith Walk, Edinburgh EH1
3AF and by associated companies, branches and representatives
throughout the world.

First published 1986

Printed in U.S.A.

ISBN 0-443-08353-3

7 6 5 4 3 2 1

Library of Congress Cataloging in Publication Data
Main entry under title:

Hand rehabilitation.

   (Clinics in physical therapy ; v. 9)
   Includes bibliographies and index.
   1. Hand—Wounds and injuries—Patients—Rehabilita-
tion. 2. Physical therapy. I. Moran, Christine A.
II. Series. [DNLM: 1. Hand. 2. Hand Injuries—
rehabilitation. W1 CL831CN v.9 / WE 830 H2327]
RD559.H3596   1986   617′.575044   85-26891
ISBN 0-443-08353-3

Manufactured in the United States of America

Contributors

Patricia L. Baxter, O.T.R.
Clinical Director of Work Therapy, Hand Rehabilitation Center, Philadelphia, Pennsylvania

Anne D. Callahan, M.S., O.T.R.
Assistant Director, Therapy Department, Hand Rehabilitation Center, Philadelphia, Pennsylvania

Patricia Theiss Casler, M.A., O.T.R.
Private Practice, Manhattan Rehabilitation Group, New York, New York

Heather L. Delp, M.S., R.P.T.
Private Practice, Physical Therapy Associates, East Stroudsburg, Pennsylvania

Maureen Gateley Gribben, R.P.T.
Wichita Public School System, USD 259, Wichita, Kansas

Maureen Hardy, M.S., R.P.T.
Clinical Instructor, The Therapy Center, University of Mississippi Medical Center, Jackson, Mississippi

Ellen Ring Horovitz, M.A., R.P.T.
Private Practice, Manhattan Rehabilitation Group, New York, New York

Valerie Holdeman Lee, R.P.T.
Director, Hand Rehabilitation Associates P.C., Phoenix, Arizona

Christine A. Moran, M.S., R.P.T.
Director, The Richmond Upper Extremity Center; Assistant Clinical Professor of Physical Therapy, Medical College of Virginia, Virginia Commonwealth University, Richmond, Virginia; Adjunct Assistant Clinical Professor of Physical Therapy, Old Dominion University, Norfolk, Virginia

Sandra J. Robinson, O.T.R.
Hand Management Center of St. Joseph's Hospital, Elmira, New York

Nancy I. Rosenblum, R.P.T.
Clinical Assistant Professor of Physical Therapy, Medical College of Virginia, Virginia Commonwealth University; Private Practice, Hand Management Specialists, Richmond, Virginia

Donald G. Shurr, R.P.T.
University of Iowa Hospitals, Department of Physical Therapy, Iowa City, Iowa

Mary K. Sorenson, R.P.T.
Director of Hand Therapy, Hand Surgery and Rehabilitation Center, Washington D.C.

Preface

This volume of *Clinics in Physical Therapy* has been planned to bring together the basic and clinical sciences as they apply to hand rehabilitation. It is often very easy for a specialty to develop standard treatment programs during its early rapid growth phase and subsequently attempt to substantiate scientifically its rationale for treatment.

The goal of the authors is to present to the reader a scientific rationale for their respective treatment approaches. As the editor, I certainly was pleased to find it not necessary to encourage the authors in developing the basic science foundation of their treatment approaches. They all eagerly developed and wove that theme easily into their respective chapters.

In this volume, hand rehabilitation topics such as fracture management and tendon management are presented in a different manner than in other chapters and articles already published. Special chapters on vascular hand management, replantation, and splinting are handled in a manner to be of interest to both hand therapist and general physical therapist.

It has been well recognized that, if we are to encourage the growth of our profession and clinical specialty, our treatment of the hand patient demands a more scientific basis. These chapters were written with this thought in mind, and it is hoped that they stimulate and challenge the reader as he or she undertakes the management of the hand injured patient.

Christine A. Moran, M.S., R.P.T.

Contents

1. Preserving Function in the Inflamed and Acutely
   Injured Hand   1
   Maureen Hardy

2. Advances in Flexor and Extensor Tendon
   Management   17
   Nancy I. Rosenblum and Sandra J. Robinson

3. Sensibility Measurement and Management   45
   Christine A. Moran and Anne D. Callahan

4. Conservative Management of Vasospastic
   Diseases   69
   Heather L. Delp

5. Replantation: Current Clinical Treatment   91
   Ellen Ring Horovitz and Patricia Theiss Casler

6. The Therapist's Role in Finger Joint Arthroplasty   117
   Donald G. Shurr

7. Physical Capacity Evaluation and Work Therapy for
   Industrial Hand Injuries   137
   Patricia L. Baxter

8. The Painful Hand   147
   Valerie Holdeman Lee

9. Splinting Principles for Hand Injuries   159
   Maureen Gateley Gribben

10. Fractures of the Wrist and Hand   191
    Mary K. Sorenson

Index   227

HAND REHABILITATION

1 | Preserving Function in the Inflamed and Acutely Injured Hand

Maureen A. Hardy

> The hand is an organ, if one part is injured,
> the entire organ suffers.
> —*W. Merritt*

HAND FUNCTION

The ability to use our hands requires sensation, mobility, stability, and freedom from disabling pain or anxiety. A breakdown in any of these areas, at any location of the hand, will affect normal performance. One need only remember one's own last trivial injury, such as a fingertip burn, and how incapacitated the whole hand became. Every activity seemed to bump or aggravate that one tiny spot and caused the assumption of comical postures of protection or substitute patterns until healing was complete. More severe injuries, requiring longer healing time, also cause a change in hand function, which can range from isolated joint stiffness to a full-blown reflex sympathetic dystrophy. Considering the immobilizing effect of pain and the close interplay of parts in the hand, preserving function in all uninjured structures is unquestionably the first goal of therapy.

In the hand, successful healing does not necessarily correlate with return to function. Repaired tendons that develop normal tensile strength yet do not glide are functional failures. The decision to preserve injured parts assumes that these restored parts will contribute to hand use, rather than become useless or painful appendages. Postoperative management programs have the important requirement that they maximize function without disrupting wound healing. In order to develop rational postoperative programs we must begin with an understanding of what is scar and how it is formed.

1

HAND WOUNDS

Scar—Friend or Foe

As children we all tried to catch salamanders and were shocked as the animal pulled away to safety, leaving his leg in our grasp. The poor salamander was not doomed to a three-legged life, as he possessed the physiological capability to regenerate in full the lost limb. Evolution has bestowed many biological gifts on primates, but along the way most of our body structures lost the ability to regenerate. Select tissues such as peripheral nerve, bone, fat, and liver cells can regenerate under optimum conditions, after minimal wounds.[1] Extensive wounding to these and other structures are repaired instead through the process of scar formation.

Scar formation, also referred to as adhesions, cicatrix, and fibrosis, is our primary method of restoring tissue integrity. All wounds pass through the same sequence and mechanism of repair, yet vary markedly in the final cosmetic and functional result. Scars that close the wound, impart stability, blend cosmetically with the surrounding tissue, and allow the structure to resume its preinjury function can definitely be classified as "friends." Problem scars fall into two classifications[2]: (1) failure to heal, as seen in ischemic and scurvy conditions; (2) excessive repair, including hypertrophic scars, keloids, and contractures. Painful scars may be included in the last category if one presumes the underlying cause to be scar entrapment of terminal branches of sensory nerves.[3]

Acute trauma to the hand, such as crush injuries, will result in multiple tissue wounds. The proximity of numerous structures in the small volume of the hand adds a further complication to functional healing. Is it possible for the body's repair system to differentiate the functional needs in these varying tissues? How can we expect tendon ends to heal with a rigid scar capable of withstanding normal muscle pull and yet tissues only a few millimeters away, such as paratenon and blood vessels, to heal with minimal scar strength? Initially, the scar surrounds and invades all structures, binding them together in a single unit or one large wound.[4] As wound healing progresses, the scar "differentiates" in various tissues by means of its response to the internal and external stresses applied. Internal influences refer to the collagenolytic activity during the last stage of wound healing, when collagen is biochemically removed in some areas and deposited in others. External influences in the form of motion and directional stress affect the orientation of the scar and, thus, its physical properties.[5,6]

It is hypothesized that scar tissue takes on the characteristics of the tissue it is healing.[7] The induction theory refers to the way in which the connective tissue matures producing either dense, unyielding scar or pliable mobile scar. The problem that arises most often in the acutely injured hand is the binding together of two structures by a scar, which restricts full mobility in one of the tissues.[8] Metacarpal fractures associated with extensor tendon lesions are a perfect example of this phenomenon. The one wound phase often resolves into one scar, binding the healed bone to the repaired tendon. The scar between these two structures lying close together reflects the denser characteristics of bone and results in an osteotenodesis rendering the tendon adherent and immobile. In this example, the internal forces did not help to differentiate the bone from the tendon scar. One of the ultimate goals of wound-healing research remains the control of internal overhealing.[9] However, laboratory research on controlling and eliminating scar internally can not yet be used safely in the clinic. The current clinical challenge is to influence the type of scar formed by external means, while allowing tissue repair to proceed normally in each injured structure.

Wound Healing Stages

All wounds, whether the result of surgery or trauma, progress through the same stages toward repair. The time frames given reflect normal, uncomplicated healing. Infections, edema, and the use of steroids are examples of factors that prolong certain stages. Management protocols must be flexible enough to recognize complications, if present, and to adjust the timing of therapeutic intervention (Table 1-1).

I. Inflammatory Phase (0–3 Days).   At the time of wounding, a vascular reaction takes place locally to stop the blood flow. Injured vessels initially contrict for a short period. Mast cells within the injured connective tissue later release histamine, a vasodilator. The now dilated vessels allow more blood to pass into the injured area at a rapid rate, maintaining the blood's high temperature.[10] The inflamed part is thus warmer and redder than normal. Vasodilation also allows leakage of plasma into the wound area, creating an edematous exudate. This results in the clinical picture of inflammation, characterized by redness, swelling, heat, and pain. The pain is probably due to the injury itself and pressure on sensory nerves in the injured area.[11]

Edema fluid in the extremities varies in its composition. The factors responsible for initiating the tissue effusion are also responsible for the type of fluid formed. Edema, caused by increased hydrostatic pressure in semipermeable but undamaged capillaries, is low in protein content and is termed "transudate."[12] Congestive heart failure, hepatic or kidney pathology, and venous stasis result in a lymphedema that is often responsive to elevation, diuretic drugs, and dietary salt restriction. In these situations the hydrostatic pressure gradient between capillary and tissue must be restored in order for the edema fluid to be reabsorbed. It is also interesting that edema low in protein produces minimal fibroplasia, that is, miminal residual scarring. Longstanding hand edema can cause poor joint positioning with residual joint contractures, but adhesions are absent.

Table 1-1. Wound Healing Stages and Management Techniques

Wound Healing Stage	Time Frame	Management
Inflammatory phase	0–3 d	Dressings
		Debridement
		Antibiotics
		Elevation
		Good nutrition
Fibroplasia phase	4 d–3 wk	Control contraction
		Gentle active motion for tensile strength acceleration
Remodelling phase	3 w–6 mo/1 yr	Dynamic or serial splints
		Active and passive mobilization
		Heat with stretch
		Electrical stimulation
		Controlled activities

Local injury to the extremity causes a disruption of capillary integrity and results in effusion high in protein content. The edema that has leaked out of the damaged vessels is called "exudate." This protein fluid is rich with fibroblasts that are not reabsorbed by the blood. Wound edema involves fluid high in protein content in which fibroplasia is prominent (Fig. 1-1).

Hemostasis eventually occurs due to platelet aggregation. Blood platelets begin to adhere to the damaged vessel walls and form a plug which stops blood flow.[13] Another clotting factor, fibrinogen, forms fibrin plugs in the locally damaged lymphatics, stopping any drainage from the injured area. This is a safety measure to contain and seal off the spread of infection.[14]

The later part of this phase involves the process of phagocytosis, ridding the wound of necrotic tissue. Leukocytes and macrophages migrate from dilated vessels into the area of injury in order to kill bacteria. The leukocytic population is short-lived in the wound, but the macrophages remain in the wound until healing is complete. It appears that the macrophage acts as a "director cell" in the following sequence of repair, releasing chemotactic substances that bring in other macrophages and stimulate the growth of fibroblasts.[15] Macrophages are the key cells of the inflammatory phase. Their elimination by anti-inflammatory steroids causes primary repair to suffer.[16] Con-

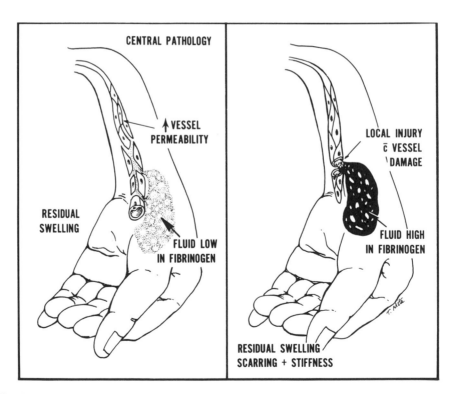

Fig. 1-1. Two types of hand edema. (Left) Transudate—low prokin effusion from semipermeable but undamaged vessels results in hand swelling but no adhesion; (right) Exudate—high protein effusion from injured vessels results in swelling, scarring, and stiffness.

versely, excessive inflammation will lead to an excessive macrophage population, stimulating greater numbers of fibroblasts to produce more collagen. The net result of prolonged inflammation is greater fibroplasia and increased scarring.[17]

The last important process that occurs during the inflammatory phase is the generation of new capillary buds reaching into the injured area. Healing cannot take place without good nourishment and oxygenation. These new vessels bridging the wound bed are "fragile and leaky,"[15] requiring immobilization of the wound to protect their delicate growth.

Management of the acutely injured hand during the first phase is directed toward assisting the cellular processes that are occurring. Debridement of necrotic tissue, evacuation of hematomas, and control of bacteria aid in decreasing the recruitment of macrophages. If the need for these inflammatory cells is minimized, then subsequent fibrosis will be minimal. Control of edema by proper elevation, notably supported elevation overnight,[18] assists in decreasing excessive swelling. The plugged, damaged lymphatics do not regenerate until the end of this phase and, therefore, cannot assist with drainage. Increased tissue exudate is a physiological stimulus to increased fiber deposition.[19] Moderate swelling is an unavoidable part of inflammation, and it is necessary to prevent the delayed healing common with wound dehydration.[20] Our goal is to prevent excessive edema with its deleterious effects, chiefly through patient education. Immobilization, proper dressings, and delicate handling of the wound will protect the fragile, newly formed capillary buds from trauma. Malnutrition prior to injury hampers the immune response. Vitamin deficiencies, especially of vitamins A and C, and protein depletion in the diet seriously affect the patient's ability to fight infection.[21] It is apparent in this phase that any factors that impede wound healing do so by increasing the risk of sepsis. Prolonged sepsis recruits more fibroblastic action in the second phase of wound healing.

II. Fibroplasia Phase (4 Days–3 Weeks). This phase of wound healing has two main goals: to resurface the wound and to impart strength. In open wounds, threads of fibrin from the original exudate form a framework of strands across the wound. At the wound surface, epithelial cells increase their mitotic rate about 40 times higher than uninjured tissue.[22] Other epithelial cells begin to migrate from the uninjured edge into the wound, following the fibrin framework as their guide. This epithelialization is maximal in moist wounds, and usually covers the surface of the wound on the third day. Coverage of the wound by epithelial cells serves the dual function of preventing fluid loss from the wound and providing a barrier against infection.[23]

The growth and migration of epithelium across the wound bed closes the superficial surface only. Below, in the granulation tissue, fibroblasts migrate into the wound area, following the same fibrin strands as did the migrating epithelial cells. These fibroblasts now become the most prominent cell type in the wound. Damaged capillaries also begin to bud and grow into the wound, forming a rich capillary network by the end of the second week. The dehydrated scab often falls off at this time, revealing a red, highly vascular scar. Early wound strength is minimal, depending on cohesive forces in the exudate, epithelial cells, and fibroblasts.[24] Until collagen fibers are produced, the wound can be easily disrupted.

Migratory fibroblasts in the wound stop their march across the bed when they meet and touch migratory fibroblasts from the other side. This cessation of movement when meeting a similar cell is called "contact inhibition." Specialized fibroblasts which have the contractile properties of smooth muscle cells have been identified within the wound. These "myofibroblasts" exert a central pull on the wound edges, which helps to decrease the size of the wound. This contraction process is a normal mechanism for minimizing the area to be healed.[25] If the wound is in an area character-ized by abundant, loose skin and immobile deeper structures, then contraction will as-sist healing with minimal deformity. This is not the case in the hand, however. Here we have numerous mobile structures covered by adherent palmar skin and dorsal skin which must possess enough redundancy to permit full fist closure. Small, approxi-mated hand wounds do not require extensive or prolonged contraction for healing. But open hand wounds allowed to heal by contraction pull the tissues in the direction of the wound. The underlying joints, also, are pulled in this direction by their tissue attach-ments. It is known that joints held immobile will develop secondary changes in their periarticular connective tissue.[26] The fixed, rigid joints that develop give the clinical picture known as joint "contracture." It is important to differentiate these two pro-cesses: *contraction*, a normal biological event which occurs during wound healing; and *contracture*, secondary fixed joint stiffness.[25]

Because joint contractures are a sequel to uncontrolled contraction in open hand wounds, proper management must be initiated early. Studies have shown that the forces for contraction can be diminished through the use of thick skin grafts and splinting used in combination. Various types of skin grafts help to diminish the percent of wound contraction but do not entirely inhibit the process. Split-thickness grafts are effective in diminishing contraction by 31 percent, while full-thickness grafts reduce the process by 55 percent.[27] The combined use of early grafting with splinting inhibits wound contraction by 77 percent.[28]

The fibroblasts which migrated into the wound bed have proliferated and are now ready to perform their main function, production of collagen for wound strength. About the fourth to fifth day post-injury, the local wound environment stimulates the fibroblasts to excrete tropocollagen, a weakly hydrogen-bonded molecule composed of three helical chains. Tensile strength of tropocollagen is low, and it is soluble in saline solutions.[22] Cross-links develop between the three chains in the helix, which produce a very stable, insoluble fiber known as collagen. Tensile strength develops rapidly, but at 3 weeks still has less than 15 percent of its ultimate strength.[24] The wound can now tolerate the forces of active motion without fear of wound dehiscence. In fact, external stress on the healing wound assists in the development of significantly greater tensile strength than unstressed wounds.[5] The principle that early, controlled motion has a beneficial effect on strength development was proposed decades ago by Mason and Allen.[29] Recent investigations continue to support the idea that cellular activity at the repair site is promoted by early, controlled mobilization.[6]

Controlled mobilization refers to the proper positioning, movement, and amount of force placed on a healing structure. Protocols of movement vary for different tis-sues, but all are aimed toward regaining mobility while preserving tissue integrity.

When collagen production fills the wound, the fibroblast population diminishes and finally disappears from the wound. The wound can now be judged as clinically healed, but the most important developments related to function have yet to occur.

III. Remodelling Phase (3 Weeks – 6 Months/1 Year).   In order for healing to be complete, the mass of scar tissue produced during the second stage must develop both the tensile strength and the proper configuration to allow the return of normal function. The following remodelling processes continue for 6 months to 1 year after injury.

Due to the accelerated rate of collagen production in the fibroplasia phase, the wound will have its greatest mass around the third week. The newly formed collagen appears as a gel due to its weak, soluble structure. This gel is composed of fragile, randomly-arranged collagen fibrils with low tensile strength. As the collagen fibril matures, it forms *intra*molecular cross-links between its own chains and *inter*molecular cross-links with other collagen fibrils. The resultant collagen fibers are insoluble and contribute to the progressive strengthening of the wound.[14] After 3 weeks, the total collagen content of the wound stabilizes, yet collagen synthesis is still above normal. In order for the amount of collagen in the wound to remain at a constant level, with high synthesis occurring, it is inevitable that destruction of collagen must now be occurring simultaneously. The enzyme responsible for this collagen lysis is collagenase. In optimum conditions, collagen production is balanced by collagen lysis, and the wound is in equilibrium. Pathological factors that tip this scale in either direction can cause increased lysis with wound disruption (as seen in scurvy, Marfan's disease, and Ehlers-Danlos syndrome) or can suppress lysis (which leads to hypertrophic scarring and keloids). The rapid, ongoing production of new collagen and removal of the old is part of the biological mechanism of scar remodelling. Obviously, clinical methods employed to influence the characteristics of the newly formed collagen will have their greatest effect at this stage of high collagen turnover, before the wound fully matures.

There is another development occurring, which has direct influence on scar remodelling and tensile strength. Initially, the collagen fibrils are deposited throughout the wound in a random fashion of disorganization. As cross-linking is happening, orientation of the fibers begins to change the architecture of the wound. Scar fibers begin to organize and form different weaves in different tissues. Our "one wound concept" of similar scar uniting all injured structures is about to change.

As the wound heals, it begins to receive some of the stresses and strains normal to the surrounding tissue. Collagen fibers respond to tension by lining up in parallel fashion along the lines of tension.[15] Tensiometric studies on paired wounds[30] with and without applied tension, show that unstressed wounds are composed of randomly arranged fibers with lower tensile strength. Those wounds that healed under tension showed parallel orientation of fibers and were twice as strong as their counterparts.

It appears that the collagen molecule, through a change in its pattern or weave, attempts to remodel to resemble the pre-injury condition. Scar adjacent to bone, between cut tendon ends, or in thick fascia, purposely reorganizes to form a thick, dense weave capable of withstanding high stress. Conversely, scar formed near skin, paratenon, and blood vessels maintains a loose weave characteristic of these tissues. Thus, tension transmitted through the wound, plus the surfaces against which the wound forms, are factors responsible for inducing the remodelling of scar.[24]

The physiological process of remodelling does not always result in restoration of normal hand function. Edema, prolonged immobilization, infection, and massive tissue injury result in greater fibroplasia with a resultant larger mass of collagen to be remodelled. The amount of scar to be remodelled is inversely related to the return of hand function. Attempts to control molecular bonding and the equilibrium of collagen synthesis and degradation through pharmacological means remains at the laboratory level. Research in wound healing has made great strides and may someday aid in discovering how to ultimately heal without scar.[31] For the present, our most effective means of clinically affecting the remodelling of collagen is through understanding of the biological processes occurring and applying the proper stress at the proper time. Since this is the most important phase for regaining function, the rest of this chapter will focus on rehabilitative methods to remodel scar tissue.

THE ART AND SCIENCE OF REMODELLING SCAR TISSUE

Hand therapy is "behavioral modification of the fibroblast during the healing response."

—Weber and Davis

The above definition expresses our attempts as therapists to favorably influence the healing tissue through our procedures. But wound healing is a dynamic process passing through several stages. Consequently, the same procedure applied in one stage could result in improved function, yet, inappropriately applied in another stage, could contribute to increased scarring. A slight alteration of the above definition, in recognition of these facts, would state, "behavioral modification of the fibroblast during the *appropriate* healing phase."

The Science

During the first two phases of healing, we were primarily concerned with providing an optimum environment for the healing processes. Our only intervention into wound dynamics was to minimize contraction in large wounds to prevent deforming contractures. The time is now right to begin "molding" the scar for the desired outcome.

A good analogy is to consider the mass of scar just produced as if it were newly poured concrete (Fig. 1-2). It is impossible to leave an imprint on liquid concrete when it is first poured. The cement is too fluid at this point and cannot maintain any indentations. If you were to vigorously attempt to mark the cement, the result would probably be cement spewed everywhere. Vigorous therapy used too early in the healing process can incite inflammation and edema, or it can even disrupt the wound. We must time our procedures to coincide with the right stage. When concrete reaches just the right consistency, it is moldable. Children delight in walking through the soft, viscous substance, leaving their initials to be hardened permanently. The wound entering the remodelling phase is similar to concrete beginning to set. It is strong enough to withstand stress and will deform directionally in response to it. Whatever we do, or fail to do, at this point will become permanent as the cross-linking terminates and the wound fully matures. Late attempts to prevent joint and skin contractures, to gain range of motion

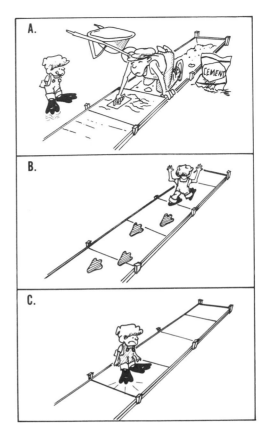

Fig. 1-2. Scar Remodelling. (A) Early scar is too weak to respond to directional stress. (B) Properly timed stress to cross-linking collagen results in favorable scar remodelling. (C) stress applied for late to matured collagen has no effect.

and tendon gliding are as frustrating as the child who arrives to play in the concrete too late. It is set now and will not permit any imprints.

The skeptic should now rightfully ask whether there is any research data to support the above analogy. Arem and Madden[32] hypothesized that stress could modify scar morphology if the forces were applied at a select time. Rats with bilateral incisions received magnetic tension to one side alone. The unstressed side served as a control. The animals were divided into two treatment groups: the first received their initial experimental stress 3 weeks after wounding; the second group were held until 14 weeks post-surgery before being subjected to tension. Their results showed that tension on internal scar had no effect on the rate of collagen synthesis or lysis. Examination of the scar complex revealed the exciting results of remodelling. The scar formed under tension initiated at 3 weeks was markedly elongated, with collagen fibers oriented in the direction of tension. The unstressed (control) scar from the same animal was tightly approximated, with random orientation of collagen fibers. Interestingly, the second group of rats, which received their tension beginning at 14 weeks, revealed scar tissue similar in appearance and form to the unstressed control side. It appears from this data that old scar is not amenable to physical changes, i.e., it does not remodel. The young, immature scar can be altered morphologically by stress and remodelled in direct response to that stress, producing lengthened, attenuated adhesions. The two parameters of time and direction of stress are our guideposts when attempting to remodel scar clinically.

Other body tissues have been studied as to their response to stress and remodelling capabilities. Bora[33] found that repaired nerves adjust to tension by increasing their compliance and cross-sectional area. Thus, peripheral nerves can remodel to properly timed stress to permit functional joint excursion. Lengthening of bone through distraction methods are now used clinically to increase digital length.[34] Tendon repair presents a challenge in both the timing and techniques of mobilization. Remodelling of repaired tendons must permit gliding, while not disrupting the injured portion. Numerous studies[35-37] on tendon scar tissue demonstrate that lengthened adhesions about the repaired site will permit gliding, which can be achieved by controlled early mobilization. Postoperative management protocols for MP joint implants[38] are based on similar remodelling principles. Splints and exercises are directed towards elongation of dorsal and volar capsule scar tissue, in order to permit flexion and extension; yet the scar formed laterally about the implant is unstressed in order to assure tight support against deformation.

Houck[39] demonstrated that not only is the injured area subjected to remodelling forces, but adjoining, non-injured tissues change their collagen production rate also in response to inflammation. Since collagen turnover is accelerated in normal tissues proximal to an injured area, uninjured structures can become fixed in nonfunctional positions if left immobile during healing. Treatment regimes must also be directed to maintaining uninjured tissue mobility during healing of wounds.

We have sufficient data to support the premise that prolonged stress on a new scar will cause reorganization of collagen. Our goal in rehabilitation of hand injuries is twofold: to know the desired outcome for the involved tissue and to choose procedures that will properly affect those tissues.

The Art

When scientific research reveals new data on hand injuries and healing, we must accept the challenge of revamping our protocols in accordance with this new information. However, treatments based only on the current accumulation of scientific data would limit the rehabilitation potential of most patients. The art of hand therapy incorporates the skill and insights which long years of experience and inquiry into the techniques of therapy have produced. As specialists, we must clarify what we do and why we do it, and if we don't know why something works, we must state the problem and continue to investigate.

Artistic works are usually appreciated subjectively, without one's having to validate their design. Although many rehabilitation procedures lack scientific research support, therapists can attempt to confirm their effects through objective measurements following the treatment. Consider first the structure to be remodelled, and choose an objective parameter to measure, such as passive joint motion for capsular stiffness; active finger-tip to distal palmar crease distance for tendon gliding; volumetrics for edema. Next choose the mode by which to act directly upon the involved structure, by joint mobilization for capsular stiffness; by electrical stimulation for tendon gliding; by activities in elevation for edema. Following the treatment, remeasure the structure, and compare this value with your initial findings. If no change is evident over a short period of time, then the above sequence must be re-evaluated as to its correct design. Effective remodelling results in improved objective measurements.

One study[40] developed a sequential evaluation-treatment-evaluation protocol for stiff joints, which aided in the selection and modification of hand therapy. Their program results showed that 87 percent of the stiff joints responded favorably and did not require surgery.

Complex hand injuries may cause many problems; therefore, they must be carefully evaluated, and priorities must be established. Attempting to affect all structures simultaneously can overwhelm the patient and result in poor compliance or overwhelm the hand, resulting in exacerbation of inflammation. This principle is often violated by complex splints designed to affect all joints concurrently. Compliance will be better achieved by several simple splints, each with a separate function.

Our primary goal is always to maintain normal mobility in uninjured tissues. Control of edema and pain are necessary in order that all tissues may tolerate our remodelling stresses.[41] "The hand that hurts will not work" is a basic tenet to remember.[11] The use of TENS, Neuroprobe, massage, fluidotherapy, and desensitization techniques are examples of modalities used for pain control.

Heat combined with a load producing elongation of connective tissue has some scientific support.[42,45] No heat modality has been shown to be superior in affecting this tissue extensibility.[43] Clinical applications of heat can easily be modified to permit simultaneous stretching of the scar (Fig. 1-3). The elongation of the scar produced in a therapy session will not become permanent until the scar biology has a chance to remodel the collagen through its synthesis and destruction cycle. Therefore, initial gains must be maintained for a period of time in order to permit the morphological restructuring to take place. Dynamic and serial splints are an ideal method for preserving gains made in therapy, until they are permanently incorporated into the tissue structure.

Passive mobilization affects joint capsular structures, but only active motion will affect tendon gliding. Electrical stimulation can be used to encourage tendon gliding, while also pulling on restrictive adhesion. Biofeedback devices aid the patient in focusing his active exercises on the tissues requiring stress.[44]

SUMMARY

The formation of a scar in response to injury is a normal biological process necessary for healing. All wounds progress through the stages of initial inflammation, which in turn induces fibroblastic production of collagen. As the collagen matures in the final stage, it is amenable to remodelling forces.

During the first two stages of healing, therapy is directed towards assisting the biological sequence of repair. By minimizing edema and sepsis, the therapist allows these initial phases to conclude quickly.

The effects of remodelling can be seen in the newly formed collagen, as well as in surrounding uninjured structures. If remodelling takes place without planned direction, the entire hand can be left crippled by adherent tendons, joint stiffness, and contracted

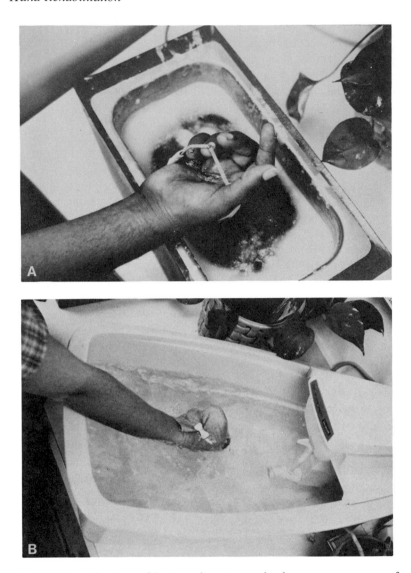

Fig. 1-3. Clinical applications of heat can incorporate simultaneous stress to scar for tissue elongation. (A) Paraffin with rubber band traction to finger-nail hooks. (B) Ace wrap utilized in whirlpool.

soft tissues. It is our challenge to understand the scar characteristics desired in each structure and appropriately to choose the modality of treatment that will affect this scar. Clinical methods do exist which can aid in directing the remodelling of scar tissue.

Remodelling will be most successful when the patient can actively use both hands again as he re-enters his preinjury life style. The ability to resume one's career, enjoy one's hobbies, and care for one's personal needs should be the final and only remodelling forces necessary.

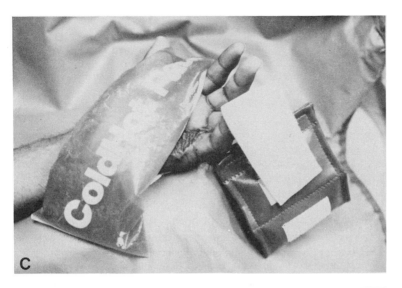

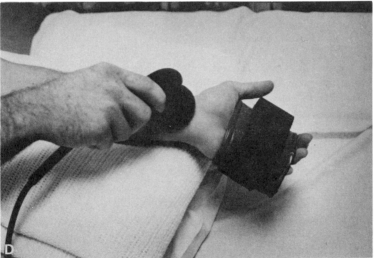

Fig. 1-3 (*cont.*) (C) Hot packs on scar, with sandbag weights. (D) Ultrasound over scar, maintaining stress with weights.

REFERENCES

1. Peacock E, Van Winkle W: Repair of skin wounds. p. 204. In Wound Repair. WB Saunders, Philadelphia, 1976
2. Hunt T: Disorders of wound healing. World Surg 4:271, 1980
3. Defalque R: Painful trigger points in surgical scars. Anesth Analg 61:518, 1982
4. Weiner L, Peacock E: Biologic principles affecting repair of flexor tendons. Adv Surg 5:145, 1971
5. Sussman M: Effect of increased tissue traction upon tensile strength of cutaneous incisions in rats. Proc Soc Exp Biol Med 123:38, 1966

6. Gelberman R et al: Effects of early intermittent passive mobilization on healing canine flexor tendons. J Hand Surg 7(2):170, 1982

7. Repair of tendons and restoration of gliding function. p. 367. In Peacock E, Van Winkle W (eds): Wound Repair. WB Saunders, Philadelphia, 1976

8. Weeks P, Wray C: Bone regeneration and articular cartilage repair. p. 25. In Management of Acute Hand Injuries. 2nd Ed. CV Mosby, St Louis, 1978

9. Cohen K, McCoy B: The biology and control of surface overhealing. World Surg 4:3:289, 1980

10. Hambury H et al: The use of differential skin temperature measurements in the evaluation of post-traumatic oedema control. Med Biol Eng 13(2):202, 1975

11. Jabaley M, Curtis R: Hand injuries. In Hardy JD (ed): Rhoads Textbook of Surgery. 5th Ed. JB Lippincott, Philadelphia, 1977

12. Witte C, Witte M: Significance of protein in edema fluid. Lymphology 4:29, 1971

13. Flynn M, Rovee D: Promoting wound healing. Am J Nurs 82(10):1543, 1982

14. Bryant M: Wound healing. Clin Symp 29:3, CIBA Pharmaceutical Co, Summit, NJ, 1977

15. Hunt T, Van Winkle W: Wound healing: Normal repair. Fundamentals of Wound Management in Surgery. Chirurgecom Publ, South Plainfield, NJ, 1976

16. Leibovich S, Ross R: The role of macrophages in wound repair. Am J Pathol 78(1):71, 1975

17. Linsky C et al: In Dineen P, Hildick-Smith G (eds): The surgical wound. Lea & Febiger, Philadelphia, 1981

18. Eccles M: Hand volumetrics. Br J Phys Med, 18:5, 1956

19. Absoe-Hansen G et al: Tissue edema—A stimulus of connective tissue regeneration. J Invest Dermatol 32:505, 1959

20. Peacock E, Van Winkle W: The biochemistry and the environment of wounds and their relation to wound strength. p. 145. In Peacock E, Van Winkle W (eds): Wound Repair. WB Saunders, Philadelphia, 1976

21. Burke J: Infection. Fundamentals of Wound Management in Surgery. Chirurgecom Inc, South Plainfield, NJ, 1977

22. Hugo N: General aspects and healing of skin. p. 339. In Kernahan D, Vistnes L (eds): Biological Aspects of Reconstructive Surgery. Little, Brown and Co, Boston, 1977

23. Peacock E, Van Winkle W: Contraction. p. 54. In Wound Repair, WB Saunders, Philadelphia, 1976

24. Madden J: Wound healing: The biological basis of hand surgery. Clin Plast Surg 3(1):3, 1976

25. Rudolph R: Contraction and the control of contraction. World J Surg 4:279, 1980

26. Akeson WH et al: Collagen cross-linking alterations in joint contractures: Changes in the reducible cross-links in peri-articular connective tissue collagen after nine weeks of immobilization. Connect Tissue Res 5:15, 1977

27. Stone P, Madden J: Biological factors affecting wound contraction. Surg Forum 26:547, 1975

28. Sawhney C, Monga H: Wound contraction in rabbits and the effectiveness of skin grafts in preventing it. Br J Plast Surg 23:318, 1970

29. Mason M, Allen H: The rate of healing of tendons: An experimental study of tensile strength. Ann Surg 113:424, 1941

30. Thorngate S: Effect of tension on healing of aponeurotic wounds. Surgery 44(4):619, 1958

31. Peacock E: Healing and control of healing—introduction. World J Surg 4:269, 1980

32. Arem A, Madden J: Effects of stress on healing wounds: I. Intermittent noncyclical tension. J Surg Res 20:93, 1976

33. Bora F et al: The biomechanical responses to tension in a peripheral nerve. J Hand Surg 5(1):21 1980

34. Kessler I et al: Experience with distraction lengthening of digital rays in congenital anomalies. J Hand Surg 2(5):394, 1977
35. Wray R et al: Effect of stress on the mechanical properties of tendon adhesions. Surg Forum 25:520, 1974
36. Potenza A: Concepts of tendon healing and repair. In AAOS Symposium on Tendon Surgery in the Hand, CV Mosby, Philadelphia, 1974
37. Strickland J, Glogovac S: Digital function following flexor tendon repair in zone II: A comparison of immobilization and controlled passive motion techniques. J Hand Surg 5:537, 1980
38. Madden J, DeVore G: A rational postoperative management program for metacarpophalangeal joint implant arthroplasty. J Hand Surg 2(5):358, 1977
39. Houck J: The chemistry of local dermal inflammation. J Invest Dermatol 36:451, 1961
40. Weeks P et al: The results of non-operative management of stiff joints in the hand. Plast Reconstr Surg 61(1):58, 1978
41. Prendergast K: Therapists management of a mutilated hand. p. 156. In Hunter J, Schneider L, Mackin E, Bell J (eds): Rehabilitation of the Hand. CV Mosby, St Louis, 1978
42. Warren C et al: Elongation of rat tail tension: Effect of load and temperature. Arch Phys Med Rehabil 52:465, 1971
43. Gersten J: Effect of ultrasound on tendon extensibility. Am J Phys Med 34:362, 1955
44. Brown DM et al: Feedback goniometers for hand rehabilitation. Am J Occup Ther 33(7):458, 1979
45. Warren CG: The use of heat and cold in the treatment of common musculoskeletal disorders. p. 115. In Kessler R, Hertling D (eds): Management of Common Musculoskeletal Disorders, Harper & Row, New York, 1983.

2 | Advances in Flexor and Extensor Tendon Management

Nancy I. Rosenblum
Sandra J. Robinson

Tendon injuries continue to be among the most difficult surgical and rehabilitation management problems. It is essential that the management of the hand with a tendon injury be based on a clear understanding of the principles of wound healing and on a thorough knowledge of the anatomical structures involved.

In 1941, Mason and Allen[1] stated, "Despite a great number of experimental and histologic studies which have appeared during the past 30 or more years, there is still a lack of agreement concerning even the tissues which take part in the process." They were referring to the process of tendon healing, and that same statement can be made with accuracy today, despite numerous attempts to clarify how a tendon heals. Scientists began the search for an answer to this question well before the start of the twentieth century.

The unanswered questions provide the stimulus and the challenge for the development of rational treatment programs for these injuries. The therapist and surgeon involved in the care of the person who has suffered tendon injury must extrapolate pertinent information from the available research results, consider the variables of the particular injury, and realistically assess the patient's ability to comply with a program, before an appropriate course of management can be established. The importance of each of these components cannot be overstated. In addition, successful management of an individual's tendon injury hinges upon close and clear communication among surgeon, therapist, and patient from the onset of treatment thoughout the rehabilitation period.

Numerous management methods have arisen for both flexor and extensor tendon injuries, as a result of the controversy concerning tendon healing. Due to the unfortunate fact that no single method of management has proven consistently successful, the quest for improved treatment methods continues. All those involved in the care of tendon injury must take the responsibility to continually analyze why particular methods have been chosen and what qualitative and quantitative results have occurred by using these methods. This analysis with each patient should further our attempts to increase the true scientific basis of hand therapy.

This chapter discusses advances in both flexor and extensor tendon management. It is limited to injuries treated by primary repair or repair within a few days of injury, for which no tendon grafting is required.

No attempt is made to include exhaustive descriptions of all specific management methods; rather, the focus will be on:

1.   The physiology of tendon healing and factors that affect tendon healing.
2.   The important anatomical aspects of and contrast between flexor and extensor tendons.
3.   The clinical implications and applications of these physiological and anatomical principles on management of flexor and extensor injuries.

It is the opinion of these authors that before taking the responsibility for supervising the rehabilitation process in this group of patients, the therapist must identify and understand factors that influence tendon healing. A strong basis in this area enables the therapist not only to utilize generally accepted management methods with a better understanding but also to rationally modify these techniques based on the individual injury.

TENDON HEALING: PHYSIOLOGICAL AND BIOLOGICAL PRINCIPLES

The mechanisms involved in tendon healing have been of great interest to researchers and clinicians alike. The purpose of this section is to discuss the multiple processes involved in tendon healing, as they relate to the differing philosophies of postoperative management.

A tendon's response to injury, like that of all body tissues, is dependent on its nutritional status. It is now known that a tendon has two nutritional pathways. Both vascular perfusion and synovial diffusion can support the increased metabolic requirements of a healing tendon.

Vascular Perfusion

Although it was long believed that tendons had no purposeful circulation, injection studies have now repeatedly demonstrated the vascular pattern of tendons.[2-7] Three main groups of blood vessels are described: (1) proximal vessels that enter at the musculotendinous junction, (2) intermediate vessels which enter through the meso-

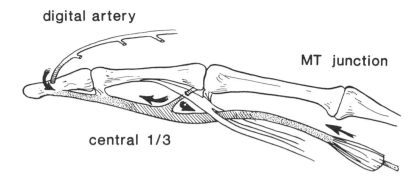

digital artery

MT junction

central 1/3

Fig. 2-1.   The segmental blood supply of a flexor tendon. The 3 main sources of nourishment are depicted: (1) musculotendinous junction, (2) vessels which enter through the mesotenon (in this flexor tendon, specialized mesotenon called "vincula" are depicted), (3) vessels at the periosteal insertion.

tenon in tendons surrounded by a sheath, (3) distally, vessels of the bone and periosteum at the periosteal insertion of the tendon[6,7] (Fig. 2-1). Peacock[6] challenged the concept that tendons can be treated as a "dead" tissue by measuring the average QO_2 for tendon to be 0.1 μ of oxygen/mg/h. This is a comparatively small metabolic rate, but enough to establish that blood vessels in tendons have a definite and vital function. Unfortunately, the blood supply is very delicate and easily interrupted when traumatized, resulting in tencocyte death and gradual collagen degradation and absorption.[6] Injection studies of tendons consistently show failure of all the vessels to fill within the suture zone.[8,9] The need is established for the formation of new blood vessels and the stage is set for a clinical predicament; adhesions can, and often do, restrict tendon gliding, yet they also contain new blood vessels carrying nutrients to the devitalized areas of the tendon.[10-13]

Although the three sources of blood supply are segmental in their nourishment capabilities,[6] together they provide what Smith describes as "uniform circulation" throughout the entire tendon.[7] The unique pattern found within the digital flexor tendon partly explains why adhesion formation has always been, and continues to be, a more frequent problem in this area. The main vascular channel is dorsally based, leaving the entire volar surface devoid of vessels.[3,5] This dorsally based system is reinforced by the vessels carried in the vincula, yet they too have a limited perfusion capacity, so that critical avascular segments have been identified in the flexor digitorum superficialis and profundus within the digital sheath[5] (Fig. 2-2A). This anatomic arrangement may offer an explanation regarding the balance between intrinsic and extrinsic healing sources — injury in an area where tendons are relatively avascular establishes a greater need for extrinsic sources of blood supply and fibroblasts, or synovial nutrition for healing.

Paratenon surrounds tendons in the forearm and proximal palm, in contrast to a synovial sheath found in the fibroosseous tunnel. Paratenon abounds in transversely oriented vessels that enter randomly into the tendon.[3] The mesotenon also supplies blood vessels that originate in a bed lying deep to the tendon and pass to its undersurface.[7,14] Therefore, tendons surrounded by paratenon have a more random and plentiful

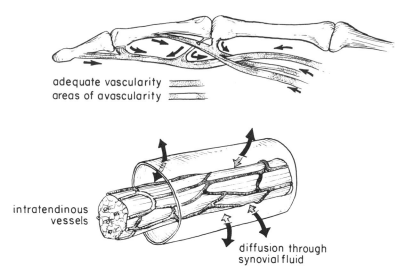

adequate vascularity

areas of avascularity

intratendinous
vessels

diffusion through
synovial fluid

Fig. 2-2. (A) The relatively avascular zones described in the digital flexor tendon. (B) The two nutrient pathways of a synovial tendon: (1) perfusion through intratendinous vessels and (2) synovial diffusion. Synovial diffusion is thought to play a critical role in the nourishment of avascular zones.

blood supply, compared to the specialized "vincula" in the digital synovial sheath. The vincula are found with varying frequency and anatomic location, and carry numerous small vessels to and from the flexor digitorum profundus FDP and flexor digitorum superficialis FDS, communicating with the intrinsic vascularization.[2-5,15] The vulnerability of the vincula, which are frequently destroyed when a lacerated flexor tendon retracts in the palm, contributes to the historically poor results with adhesion formation in the digital canal.

Synovial Diffusion

The recognition of synovial fluid as a second nutritional pathway has led to innovations in postoperative management. If a synovial tendon can be adequately nourished by synovial diffusion, then theoretically the ingrowth of cells and vessels from surrounding tissue would not be necessary. New management philosophies challenge the classic 3-week immobilization period thought necessary to allow re-vascularization through adhesions to occur.

It is generally agreed that most tendon repairs heal with good functional results, with the exception of the digital flexor tendon. [16-18] This is due to the indiscriminate nature of healing, as well as the specialized anatomy in the digital canal. This specialization includes a complicated gliding system and pulley mechanism subjected to considerable force and friction, comprised of rigid fibrous pulleys and membranous synovial components (Fig. 2-3). The synovial membrane is highly vascularized, and the friction surface of the pulleys is completely avascular.[19,20] Evidence is accumulating

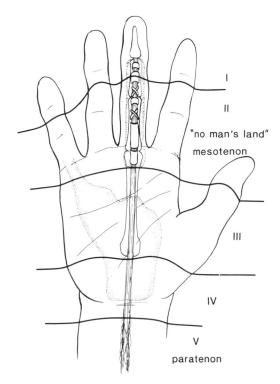

Fig. 2-3. Zones of the Hand. Note that specialized mesotenon, the vincula, are found in Zone II. Where there is no synovial sheath, the tendon is surrounded by paratenon instead, and the mechanism of vascularization is different.

that the relatively avascular zones of the pulleys, segments between vincular supply, and the volar surface of the tendon are totally, or in part, nourished by synovial diffusion. This mechanism has been likened to the system in articular cartilage. It is hypothesized that compression and decompression establish a pumping action that facilitates transport of nutrients across the synovial fluid.[5,21] If this is indeed analogous to the "specialized joint" of the digital flexor canal,[5] mobilization assumes added importance as an integral part of the mechanism of synovial diffusion.

The concept of synovial based nutrition is not entirely new. At one time, interposition membranes between a repaired tendon and the forming scar tissue were used experimentally in an effort to block adhesion formation.[11,22] This was abandoned due to the observation that flexor tendons within a sheath derive vital nutrients from the synovial fluid. Recent studies have attempted to clarify the role of synovial diffusion by looking at tendon segments detached from all vascular supply, thereby completely dependent upon synovial diffusion for survival.[23,24] Manske and associates[24] compared the uptake of tritiated proline (a radioactive tracer of collagen) in tendons detached from all vascular attachments to the uptake in segments completely separated from the synovium. Their findings of significantly less uptake in the segment isolated from the synovium defines synovial fluid as an important nutritional pathway. Regardless of which is the "primary nutrient pathway," it is our opinion that the literature supports the importance of *both* pathways, and that disruption of one alters the tendon's healing potential.

"Intrinsic versus Extrinsic" Healing

Widespread support has been gathered for three explanations as to the processes involved in tendon healing. Central to this issue is the origin of the cells responsible for this repair. Results from experimental laboratories and clinical experience show us that tendons have the capacity to heal in three ways:

1.   Extrinsic healing occurs when the paratendinous tissue and the accompanying neovascular growth supply the cells necessary for repair (Fig. 2-4A). The tendon itself is said to assume no active role.[12,13,22] In Potenza's classic study of tendon healing in dogs,[13] healing came about through the response from the sheath and ingrowth of cells

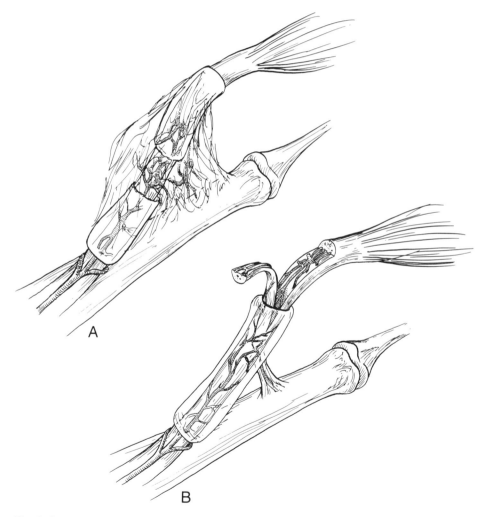

A

B

Fig. 2-4.   (A) "Extrinsic Healing" schematically drawn to show vessel-carrying adhesions. (B) "Intrinsic Healing" without the presence of adhesions.

from other surrounding tissue as a result of adhesion formation. This work was influential in establishing the belief that tendon lacked any intrinsic healing capabilities, and adhesion formation was accepted as an essential part of healing for the ingrowth of blood vessels and nutrients.

2. Intrinsic healing occurs when tendon tissue and the tendon cells participate in the healing process, without the formation of adhesions[10,21,23,25,27,28] (Fig. 2-4B). Under ideal experimental conditions, resting tenocytes have been demonstrated to transform into fibroblasts, proliferate, and synthesize collagen to participate in its own healing.[25,27,28] Lindsay and Thomson[11] observed that despite isolation from perisheath tissues, the repair process progressed at the same rate as it did in control tendons. They identified the connective tissue components of the tendon—epitenon and endotenon—as participating in the repair process. Lundborg and Rank's now well-known synovial environment model in prepateller bursa of the rabbit[23,27] supports this intrinsic healing potential. Both rabbit and human tendon segments not only remained viable, but tendon cells were observed proliferating and bridging the suture gap. Repeated later with a dialyzing membrane to prevent cell seeding from the synovial fluid, the same phenomenon was observed, further supporting the intrinsic origin and healing capabilities of the cells.

3. Healing may also occur through contributions from sources both intrinsic and extrinsic to the tendon. One source of healing does not preclude another, and it is likely that both sources are at work in varying combinations. Ketchum[30] points out that the intrinsic tendon response is often hidden beneath the massive reaction from the surrounding tissues. This is not a new idea, as Mason and Shearon in 1932[31] concluded that the tendon cells themselves begin to proliferate and participate in repair around the fourth to fifth day.

The work that demonstrates a tendon's intrinsic healing potential is exciting; unfortunately, the distance between these pure experimental models and clinical reality is far. A severed flexor tendon necessarily involves injury to several tissues in addition to the tendon—to skin, subcutaneous tissue, synovial sheath, and sometimes periosteum. Since all injured tissues will respond with an inflammatory reaction, it is difficult to imagine the real life situation where only sources intrinsic to the tendon will respond. For now, it seems necessary to accept that tendons may heal in several ways, and understanding the various factors that influence the balance between intrinsic and extrinsic sources may give us better insight into what type of healing response to expect. To quote Dr. Leonard Furlow, "It doesn't really make a difference how a tendon heals, as long as whatever does the job allows it to move!" (personal communication, May 1984)

The effects of trauma on adhesion formation are well documented.[8,9,11,32,33] Adhesions will form between the tendon and surrounding tissue at each point where the tendon surface is broken.[33] Tendon suture placed in an uninjured tendon is even enough to excite adhesion formation.[11] Berglung's work[8] revealed that the strangulating effect of the suture on the intratendinous vessels is a stimulus to adhesion formation.

Matthews and Richards investigated the effects of other factors, in addition to the original trauma, on the adherence of tendons after repair.[32] Splinting, suture, and sheath excision were evaluated separately and in various combinations. They found that with just one of the variables imposed, healing occurred without adhesion formation. Combining any two of the variables, the tendon was observed to heal partly by processes intrinsic to the tendon, augmented by extrinsic healing through adhesions. Matthews and Richards differentiated as mild and transient adhesions that tended to absorb or remodel to allow gliding of the repaired tendon. It was the combination of all three variables simultaneously that led to a massive adhesive response and a suppression of the intrinsic repair potential. They concluded that adhesions are not an essential part of the healing process of tendons, but rather a result of external factors imposed by the technique of repair and management.

Much has been written for the hand surgeon regarding techniques of repair that most favorably influence tissue response: (1) delicate handling of the tendon, (2) adoption of a suture method so as not to compromise the intrinsic vessels, (3) placement of the repair in an undamaged portion of the sheath, when possible, and (4) repair of the sheath in light of the recent emphasis on synovial nutrition. The therapist should also know the factors involved in each individual case that will influence the healing process. He or she should know whether the injury was clean or untidy, the exact location of the laceration with regard to blood supply, whether the sheath was excised, and whether the tendon retracted in the proximal palm with resultant disruption of the vincula. Responsible therapists must also be aware of procedures in their management that could favorably or unfavorably influence tissue response. Armed with this knowledge, we have a better chance of guiding the formation of favorable adhesions, for a better functional result following tendon repair.

Phases of Tendon Healing

Three phases of wound repair are generally described for all body tissue, and the reader is referred to Hardy's chapter in this volume for a more comprehensive discussion. Select concepts are discussed here to highlight their significance in tendon management.

During the early stages of healing, a single wound develops, which contains all the exposed, injured tissue within one scar.[34] This "one wound–one scar" concept is important to the time line associated with regaining motion in a newly repaired tendon. In the early stages, all injured tissues react with inflammation and celluar proliferation that results in a single fibrous scar that binds all the tissues together. As Hardy describes, a second peak in tensile strength is reached around the twenty-first day, as cross-linking of collagen molecules begins.[12,24] The strength of the union is now not only enough to withstand gentle active motion, but the tendons allowed a controlled amount of mobilization will gain tensile strength more rapidly than their immobilized counterparts.[1,35] The development of tensile strength during the period of fibroplasia is not usually a problem — the remodeling of this single scar to allow a functional degree of tendon excursion commonly is![12,32,34] This demands that, during the secondary remodeling phase, different physical properties develop within the same scar.[34] The collagen fibers between the coapted tendon ends must organize in parallel alignment in order to impart tensile strength, while the fibers along the longitudinal surface of the tendon must "disorganize" in a random orientation to allow the tendon to glide. No doubt this is why Peacock describes this secondary remodeling phase as unique to tendons.[34] Rehabilitation efforts must be directed towards both of these goals. Although an abnormally large amount of scar tissue can restrict motion, it is most often the physical characteristic of the scar that is the limiting factor.[1,32,34,36] Although the exact mechanism of remodeling is not known, elongation of the entire adhesion is thought to occur through gradual slipping of the subunits, the collagen fibers and fibrils, as they are subjected to stress.[34,37] As the scar matures, and cross-linking continues, the potential for remodeling decreases. Therapists, then, must gauge their treatment based on their "mind's eye" as to what is happening in the phases of tendon healing.

DIFFERENCES BETWEEN FLEXOR AND EXTENSOR TENDON HEALING

Both the physiology of tendon healing and the factors which effect tendon healing have been examined. However, upon close inspection, it is apparent that the healing processes and factors influencing these processes may not be identical for flexor and extensor tendons.

Mason and Allen,[1] in their study of the rate of healing tendons, cut and sutured flexor and extensor tendons of dogs. The restoration of tendon continuity was followed by examining the development of tensile strength of the union at similar time intervals. They found that the tensile strength of the flexor tendons increased more rapidly than that for the extensor tendons. The tensile strength curve of wound healing was similar for both flexors and extensors but progressed at a slower pace in the healing extensors. The only factor identified as responsible for this difference in tensile strength was the holding power of the tendon for the sutures. This suture holding power diminished more rapidly in the extensors after repair, when compared to the flexors, and was not regained as rapidly in the extensors. The authors state that this may be a phenomenon of extensor tendons in general, or it may be due to their inability to adequately immobilize the dog's foot. They did not study the actual wound healing processes of the tendons considered; therefore they can only hypothesize the cause of the differences. Caution must be exercised in the interpretation of these findings and its relevance to the digital flexors and extensors, as Mason and Allen examined not finger but wrist flexor and extensor tendons. This does not negate the importance of their findings as evidenced by the many management techniques that utilize Mason and Allen's tendon healing times as a basis for the length of immobilization following tendon repair.[36,38,39] Direct correlations, however, should be made with caution, due to the anatomical differences in the wrist and finger flexors and extensors.

The physiological processes involved in tendon healing may vary, depending on the anatomical features surrounding the tendon injured. For example, a factor that may effect a difference between the healing process of flexors and extensors is the presence or absence of a synovial sheath. The digital flexors are encased by a synovial sheath throughout most of their length (Fig. 2-5A). In contrast, the extensor tendon mechanism of the hand is extra-synovial except at the wrist, where a sheath adds protection and free gliding beneath the dorsal carpal ligament[40] (Fig. 2-5B). This anatomical difference may be of great importance since the synovial sheath has been implicated as having an important role in providing synovial fluid nutrition in flexor tendon healing,

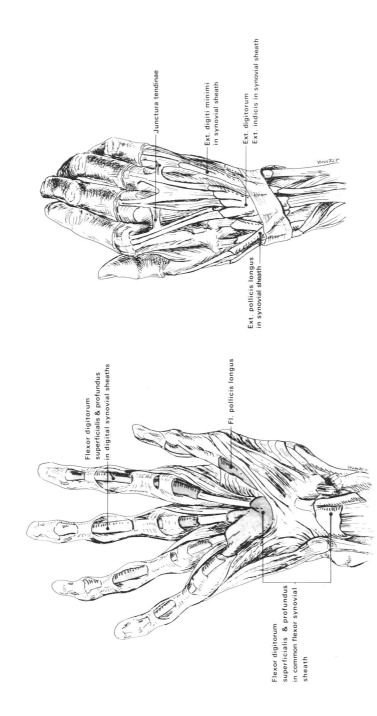

Junctura tendinae

Ext. digiti minimi
in synovial sheath

Ext. digitorum
Ext. indicis in synovial sheath

Ext. pollicis longus
in synovial sheath

Flexor digitorum
superficialis & profundus
in digital synovial sheaths

Fl. pollicis longus

Flexor digitorum
superficialis & profundus
in common flexor synovial
sheath

Fig. 2-5. (A) Volar surface of the hand showing synovial sheaths surrounding the flexor tendon. (B) Dorsal surface of the hand showing extent of synovial sheaths surrounding the extensor tendons.

especially when the vascular system of the tendon has been damaged.[23,41] We are aware of the existence of this particular anatomical difference, however, we are not at this point able to base any definite management techniques on this knowledge. When the role of synovial nutrition in tendon healing is more clearly understood, this anatomical difference may clarify the differences in healing between flexors and extensors and may influence the development of new mobilization management techniques.

As previously discussed, the blood supply of a tendon is another factor that may influence the rate and process of the tendon repair. Specifically, flexor tendons within their sheath, receive blood supply from long and short vincula and are avascular in some areas. In contrast, the extensors are supplied in their asynovial areas by arteries that pass freely through loose connective tissue. In the carpal region where extensors are enclosed by synovial sheaths, their supplying vessels traverse the mesotenon. These are not, however, specialized mesotenon (vinculae), as seen in the flexors.[42] It is a reasonable assumption, based on the nature of their vascularity, that the extensor tendons may be less prone to total devascularization than the flexor tendons. A tendon repaired with clean bleeding ends undoubtedly is more likely to heal after repair than a devascularized tendon repair.

Such detailed information may at times seem to have more academic value than clinical relevance. A therapist with a working knowledge of tendon anatomy and physiology will be better able to identify factors in individual injuries that will affect the management and outcome of the tendon injury. When a patient is referred with a new tendon injury, questions should immediately arise, such as: What specific tendon(s) were injured and repaired? At what level was the tendon injured, and what are the anatomical features at that level which may influence healing and/or management? What was the extent of damage, i.e., were the tendon ends clean and bleeding or were the ends crushed with no apparent vascularity? If the tendon was injured in an area enclosed by tendon sheath, was the sheath repaired?

There are numerous other important considerations, such as the age of the injured person; however, the answers to the above questions should lead the therapist to a rationale for the best management for each individual patient. Routine management methods may become less popular as more is understood about tendon healing. Specific clinical applications will be discussed in the sections to follow.

EXTENSOR TENDON MANAGEMENT

General Considerations

Injuries to the extensor tendons of the hand are often regarded lightly, but are responsible for large numbers of permanent partial disabilities and for time lost from the job.[43] Historically, the seriousness of these injuries has been and continues to be underestimated, despite the clear warnings and sage advice of many surgeons, including Bunnell, Entin, Littler, Tubiana, and Verdan.[40]

There are several feasible explanations for this apparent lack of concern for these potentially devastating injuries. First, extensor tendons are located superficially. Dorsally, they are protected only by skin and a small amount of soft tissue. Therefore, the cut tendon ends are often readily accessible, and repairs are frequently undertaken by emergency room staff who are not always aware of the most appropriate forms of postoperative management. Simple approximation of tendon ends in these complex structures, without thoughtful consideration of the postoperative care, can lead to major complications, which would otherwise be preventable with proper management.

Second, recovery from extensor tendon injury and repair, in general, has been thought by most to have a better prognosis than recovery from flexor tendon injury, since there is no fibro-osseous tunnel to encourage the formation of adhesions.[44]

Third, because extensor tendon injuries are not often associated with major nerve damage such as that so often encountered with flexor tendon injuries, the extensor tendon injuries are often deceptively regarded as simple.

The final explanation for this seeming lack of concern for these injuries is based on function. Some authors[45] contend that extension of the fingers is not as critical as flexion. They state, "Minor losses of extension are not as noticeable as losses of flexion, especially flexion at the proximal interphalangeal joint." This is perhaps true for most patients, however, a piano player or a violinist might take strong exception to this generalization.

All of these explanations, however, do not justify regarding these injuries as minor. The functional limitations resulting from these injuries are often very serious. For this reason, extensor tendon injuries require a careful and well thought out management plan.

A postoperative program for a primarily repaired extensor tendon should be aimed at regaining tensile strength of the union, gliding of the entire tendon,[12] and maintaining or restoring joint mobility. One of these elements without the others will not result in a functional repair. Postoperative care should be directed toward a balance between adequate tensile strength and gliding of the repaired tendon to achieve optimal function. The management methods chosen must allow the restoration of both elements, while not compromising uninjured portions of the hand.

A treatment plan to manage extensor tendon injury must consist of a well-conceived immobilization phase, as well as a mobilization phase. In general, the immobilization period allows the repair to regain tensile strength, while the mobilization period of management serves to both continue increasing tensile strength of the union[1,12] and to restore normal gliding of the repaired tendon. Any joint mobility lost during immobilization should be restored as close to normal as possible during the mobilization period.

The duration and position of immobilization, as well as the portion of the hand immobilized varies greatly, depending not only on the injury but also on the beliefs of the surgeon managing this phase of repair. Elliott[40] states that 3 weeks appears to be an adequate length of time for tendon healing, but the extensor tendon has been held longer traditionally because of the relative strength of the opposing flexors. Dargan[38] believes that the experimental basis for immobilization periods of 3 to 4 weeks following repair stems largely from the classical study of Mason and Allen.[1] In current clinical practice, however, management programs seem to be based on past clinical experience and on what surgeons and therapists were taught early in their training.

Very often, the therapist has no involvement in the management during the immobilization period. It is essential that the therapist be provided with the details of exactly how the immobilization phase of management was handled, as this will strongly affect the planning for the mobilization phase.

During the period of mobilization, secondary remodelling of the newly synthesized connective tissue in the healing tendon wound occurs. According to Peacock,[12] this secondary remodelling is the most critical factor to the development of different physical characteristics in portions of the same scar. That is, scar bridging the tendon ends reorganizes with the characteristics of tendon and the surrounding normally more areolar connective tissue reorganizes to approximate its normal state. Thus, how and when we intervene in this secondary remodelling phase of tendon healing with the mobilization period of management has an important effect on the ultimate function of the injured hand.

There are as many variations in the mobilization methods utilized with extensor tendon injuries as in the immobilization methods. The methods employed are primarily dependent upon the level of the injury and the length of time immobilized. Consideration must be given to how vigorously the hand can be moved and what techniques can safely be used to affect a positive change, i.e., improved tendon gliding and/or joint mobility. The basis for these techniques appears to be largely clinical experience, with no sound scientific base. Thus the therapist is charged with planning an intelligent rehabilitation program that may utilize many therapeutic modalities, many of which do not have an effect on secondary remodelling as observed clinically. This is a challenge that often requires intelligent persistence to result in a functional hand following extensor tendon repair.

MANAGEMENT BY LEVEL OF INJURY

Injuries to Common Extensor*

Anatomical Considerations. There are several anatomical considerations worth noting concerning the common extensor tendons at this level. Recall from Figure 2-5B that the extensor tendons are enclosed in synovial sheath for a short distance distal to the wrist. In this area there is a complex ligamentous arrangement consisting of numerous mesotendons,[46] which is covered dorsally by the dorsal carpal ligament (extensor retinaculum). In contrast, distal to the synovial sheath the extensors are surrounded by a delicate peritendinous fascia. There may not be any clinical difference in injuries at these levels since both paratenon and peritendinous fascia are mobile tissues; however, injuries directly under the extensor retinaculum may become adherent to this structure causing limited gliding of the repair.

Another anatomical feature at this level is the presence of junctura tendinae (see Fig. 2-5B). A complete laceration of the extensor tendon proximal to the junctura, involving the middle or little fingers, may produce only a slight extensor lag (inability to fully extend finger) at the metacarpophalangeal joint. The intact extensor of the ring

---

*Between distal end of radius to and including metacarpophalangeal (MP) joints).

finger can exert pull through these connections to provide deceptive MP extension of the injured finger. This clinical observation may result in a missed diagnosis and referral to therapy for splinting and/or exercise to decrease extensor lag. An awareness of this anatomical feature of the common extensors allows the therapist to treat the patient with extension splinting (a partial laceration of the extensor tendon could adequately heal with immobilization). If no improvement is noted after approximately 2 to 3 weeks of splinting, the surgeon should be consulted regarding the possibility of a full laceration and the need for surgical repair.

Immobilization Period and Techniques.   The management of a simple laceration of an extensor tendon in this area varies widely with respect to duration of immobilization, position of immobilization and the portion of the hand immobilized. The most conservative management methods immobilize the wrist and all digits in full extension for at least 3 weeks,[47] with some form of protective splinting being used for 6 weeks. In contrast, Dargan[38] advocates immobilization of the wrist and MP joints in extension for 2 weeks, during which time proximal interphalangeal (PIP) and distal interphalangeal (DIP) active exercise is encouraged. Active, full use of the hand is then taught with no further protective splinting. Stuart[48] splinted these injuries in a clinical study with the wrist and MP joints in extension, allowing free interphalangeal motion. Three groups were studied: those immobilized for 1 day, 10 days, and 3 weeks. The best results were found in the group immobilized for 10 days, the major complication of the 1-day group being extensor lag at the MP joint and the major complication of the 3-week group being stiffness and impaired flexion of the MP joints.

It becomes evident, when considering the complications incurred, that the traditionally long periods of immobilization may compromise the mobility of both injured and uninjured portions of the hand to insure the development of adequate tendon tensile strength. The effects of immobilization on uninjured joints have been documented[49,50] and are clinically encountered quite frequently. It appears likely from the work of Dargan[38] and Stuart[48] that extensor tendons at this level heal well when motion is begun after 2 weeks of immobilization. The danger in these earlier mobilization management approaches is to allow unrestricted movement before adequate collagen cross linking of the extensor tendon scar has occurred. This allows the more powerful flexor tendons to exert their force on the weak repair site, which may result in extensor lag or even rupture at the repair site. A new management method is suggested in the pages to follow, which balances this immobilization-mobilization dilemma.

Mobilization Period and Techniques.   The complications following the period of immobilization are readily revealed during an initial hand evaluation. Before beginning any therapy program, a thorough evaluation must be performed to determine joint (capsular) versus tendon (extracapsular) restrictions. For example, if, after an extensor tendon injury at the MP joint of the middle digit, the PIP joint of the same digit has 0° to 90° range of motion (ROM) with the MP joint stabilized in extension but only 0° to 50° ROM if the MP joint is flexed, the problem is extracapsular. Most likely, an adhesion of the repaired tendon to the overlying skin or underlying bone is causing the joint motion limitation. Rosenthal[51] describes the various characteristics of restricting scar of adhesions of the extensor tendons following repair at various levels. This information is very helpful in assessing the location(s) of the restriction(s), which are not always obvious.

Extensor lag of the MP joint following extensor tendon injury at this level is usually obvious immediately after removal of the immobilizing splint or cast, although it may occur gradually throughout the mobilization period. This is due to the secondary remodelling (attenuation) of the tendon scar in response to active flexion.

The therapy program should be based on the findings of the individual initial evaluation. Typically, a program begins with free active exercises placing emphasis on the prioritized problems. Numerous splints may be used, based on the individual problems and on the length of time since repair. For example, a dynamic extension splint to assist MP extension of the injured digit may be necessary if extensor lag is present. This assists the weak extensor while protecting it somewhat from the powerful flexor. At the same time, the MP joints of the uninjured digits may require flexion splinting to overcome MP collateral ligament shortening secondary to immobilization.

Each injury requires an individual program, even with injuries at the same level. The complications can be very different, depending upon the injury, the patient's own wound healing characteristics, and the methods utilized for immobilization.

New Approaches.   An attempt to reach an immobilization-mobilization balance that allows achievement of adequate tensile strength of the repaired tendon and maintainence of mobility of tendons and joints has been made with a method of early *protected* mobilization.[52] The method was designed for use with extensor tendon lacerations between the wrist and MP joints, in order to avoid both attenuation of the repair site and remodelling of the MP collateral ligaments.

The technique involves splinting immediately following primary repair, with the wrist in a simple cock up splint in comfortable extension in order to decrease the tension on the newly repaired extensor tendon. The MP joint of the injured digit is splinted in neutral or slight hyperextension, in such a manner that it is maintained in approximately 25° more extension relative to the adjacent uninjured MP joints (Fig. 2-6). The splint allows full MP flexion of the uninjured digits, very slight MP flexion of the injured digit, and full interphalangeal flexion of all digits (Fig. 2-7). Active range of motion within the confines of the splint is encouraged immediately. Because the extensor digitorum communis tendons are powered by a single muscle, splinting the injured digit, as described, should create less tension on the repaired tendon during a contraction than on its intact neighbors. In addition, the excursion of the injured tendon is limited by this method of splinting. The wrist and finger portions of the splint are worn at all times for 4 weeks, after which the finger portion is removed and the wrist protected for an additional 2 weeks. This method of management should be used only with compliant, reliable patients, since the splint is easily removable. It is advisable to check the splint at least once weekly to assure proper fit.

By utilizing this method, there may be enough "function" of the repaired tendon allowed to stimulate repair,[1] while simultaneously removing most of the tension on the repair to prevent attenuation. In addition, post-immobilization joint stiffness of the uninjured digits is reduced or eliminated as a result of allowing full active motion throughout the "immobilization" period.

This management approach potentially reduces the amount of time necessary for the entire rehabilitation process of an injury at this level. Because the immobilization and mobilization periods are combined, the extended periods of rehabilitation often required following traditional immobilization have not been found necessary. This po-

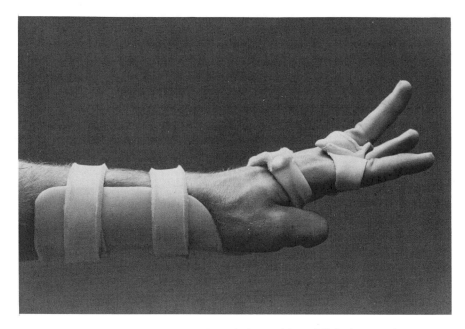

Fig. 2-6. Splint demonstrating relative position of digits in extension.

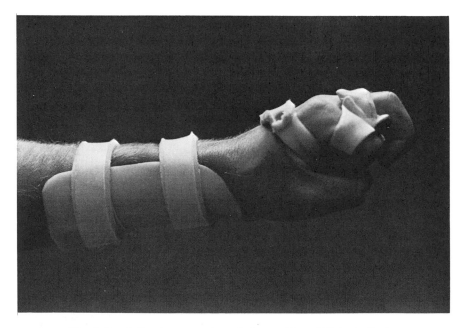

Fig. 2-7. Splint demonstrating relative position of digits in flexion.

tentially allows return to work sooner and less financial investment for the patient and/or compensation carrier. Early results of this method of management on carefully selected patients are encouraging.

Injuries to the Extensor Hood

Anatomical Considerations. Any therapist who has been called upon to treat an established boutonnière or swan neck deformity can easily appreciate the importance of proper primary treatment immediately after injury to the extensor hood. The extensor hood (apparatus, mechanism) is extremely complex. The structural complexities are made more confusing by the myriad of names given to each individual structure. Wading through the literature written about this structure can become an arduous and frustrating task if a mental list of synonyms for the various structures is not kept in mind.

A knowledge of this anatomy is essential for an understanding not only of the deformities that occur as a result of an interruption in the system, but also for an understanding of appropriate primary treatment.

Prior to discussing the immobilization or mobilization phases of treatment for primarily repaired tendon injuries at this level, a review of the anatomical structures with the commonly used synonyms should prove helpful (Fig. 2-8).

Injuries at the Proximal Interphalangeal Joint (PIP) Level. Lacerations of the extensor mechanism at the PIP joint most often disrupt the central slip and enter the joint itself. The central slip is fused with the capsule of the PIP joint.[53] This injury allows a volar displacement of the lateral bands, placing them volar to the flexion axis

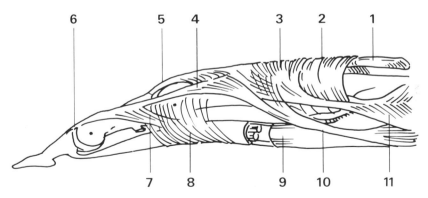

Fig. 2-8. Anatomical structures of the hand. 1. Extensor Digitorum Communis (common extensors, long extensors) 2. Sagittal Band (shroud ligaments, volar sling, laminae transversae) 3. Transverse Fibers of Interossei 4. Lateral Bands (lateral slips, lateral communis bands, lateral extensor tendons) 5. Central Slip (middle tendon, Medial extensor band or tendon) 6. Terminal Tendon (conjoined lateral bands) 7. Oblique Retinacular Ligaments (link ligament, retinaculum tendini longi, Landsmeer's ligament) 8. Transverse Retinacular Ligament 9. Fibrous Flexor Sheath 10. Lumbrical Tendon 11. Interosseous Muscle

of the joint. They become a PIP flexor and with attempted PIP extension and act to hyperextend the distal phalanx.

Any structural weakness of the extensor hood at this level allows vulnerability to the strong flexors acting on this joint. In addition, the lever arm to which the extension force is applied at the PIP joint is shorter than that for flexion which results in a mechanical advantage of the flexors at the middle phalanx.[53] Thus an injury at this level is associated with these factors which necessitate a longer period of immobilization to insure adequate collagen cross linking of the scar bridge to withstand the strong forces acting against it.

Immobilization Period. Following repair of the lacerated tendon (or the decision to utilize immobilization only to allow healing), most authors[40,44,47,52] advocate splinting for 4 to 6 weeks. Elliott[40] does point out the importance of a shorter period of immobilization in patients over 45 years of age. It is clinically observed that older patients' connective tissue is less "resilient" and therefore more prone to unyielding contractures, especially at the interphalangeal levels.

Lacerations at this level, both complete and partial, are treated by some physicians with primary suture followed by immobilization. Boyes,[54] however, believes that surgical repair is unnecessary up to 30 days following the initial injury, and advocates the use of splinting only to allow healing.

To allow healing of the lacerated tendon ends, immobilization of the injured digit with the PIP joint in full extension is necessary. Some authors[47] splint the entire injured digit in extension at all three joints in order to relieve all tension on the extensor. Most, however, immobilize the PIP joint only with splinting and/or K-wire fixation and encourage active MP and distal interphalangeal (DIP) flexion during the immobilization period. Allowing active MP flexion prevents shortening of the collateral ligaments, while allowing distal joint flexion pulls on the lateral bands, encouraging a more dorsal position at the PIP joint.[52] In addition, leaving the DIP joint free to move prevents contracture of the oblique retinacular ligament, which avoids the complication of a limitation in DIP joint flexion.

Immobilization of an injured PIP joint in the positions discussed for 4 to 6 weeks can lead to serious complications, especially when both tendon and joint are involved. Despite this fact, early mobilization has no place in the management of these injuries, due to high risk of repair rupture or attenuation. Secondary procedures for correcting failed primary procedures are difficult and most often don't provide full motion.

Mobilization Period. The management techniques utilized are dependent upon evaluation findings following immobilization. Most often there are two major concerns that guide the rehabilitation goals. The first is maintainence of tendon and joint structural continuity to prevent attenuation of the repair. The second is regaining range of motion in the PIP joint, which has had 5 weeks to become stiff in extension.

Since the flexors are much stronger than the extensor at the PIP joint, it is often wise to utilize a dynamic extension splint to assist PIP extension and resist PIP flexion for the first few weeks of the mobilization period. If any extensor lag occurs with the initiation of the therapy program, a static splint for PIP extension may be used at night to prevent further attenuation and allow the repair to remodel in a shortened position. Regaining active extension is a difficult task due to the relative weakness of the extensor and the relatively small tendon excursion.[51] Goniometric feedback utilized with extension exercises and/or activities is often helpful at this stage to encourage active use of the repaired tendon.

If, however, following immobilization, the PIP joint is so stiff in extension that no active motion is observable, the therapy program should concentrate on free active flexion. Elliot[40] believes that no flexion should be allowed for 8 weeks following the initial repair. Consideration must be given, however, to function. A finger with a PIP extension contracture is functionally very limiting, particularly if it involves the ring and little fingers.

At approximately 8 weeks following repair of the tendon, therapy can proceed to more vigorously address the problems. By this time, the new collagen bridging the tendon ends should be sufficiently cross-linked to allow gentle resistive exercises/activities in whatever direction is needed, i.e., flexion or extension. If working rigorously on flexion, it may still be necessary to utilize static extension splinting at night, as the process of secondary remodelling continues for months. With an injury at this level, taking accurate frequent range of motion measurements is essential. If the splinting program is overzealous in the direction of flexion, extension may be compromised. It is important to strike a balance and at all times keep the person's *functional* needs in mind.

Injuries at the Distal Interphalangeal Joint (DIP) Level

Lacerations or avulsions of the extensor at this level involve disruption of the terminal tendon. The DIP joint rest in a flexed posture, and active extension of the DIP is lost. The extension force normally transmitted to the DIP joint is transmitted to the PIP joint, due to the imbalance caused by disruption of the terminal tendon. With forced effort to extend the finger, hyperextension of the PIP joint will occur.

Immobilization Period. Primary injuries at this level, even if not treated for up to 2 months are often treated with immobilization alone.[47] Immobilization is most commonly maintained for 6 to 8 weeks. Although it is probably true that the tendon is "healed" after 3 weeks of immobilization, the force of the flexor digitorum profundus to pull the healing tendon apart is great. The long period of immobilization allows the tendon repair to gain enough tensile strength to withstand the strong flexor force.

Different authors suggest various positions of immobilization. Harris and Rutledge[55] demonstrated in an anatomical study that the inability to extend the distal phalanx when the PIP is flexed to 90° is due to the fact that the extensor mechanism is held distally by the central slip, and thus is checkreined. They, therefore, believe that in the treatment of a fresh laceration of the extensor at this level, the PIP joint should be splinted in flexion, with the DIP joint in full extension. This allows the central slip to pull the extensor mechanism distally and relieve any tension effects of the tendon at the DIP level, where healing of the injured tendon is occurring. In contrast, Kaplan[47] suggested immobilization of both the PIP and DIP in full extension, as he believed that it is necessary to "secure fixation of the entire dorsal apparatus with moderate relaxation of the extensor apparatus which is possible only when the finger is in the extended position at the proximal interphalangeal joint."

Both of these methods carry the danger of a severely remodelled PIP joint in the position immobilized, which may ultimately cause a more serious limitation than the original injury. PIP joint contractures can be unyielding to therapeutic measures, so thought should be given to prevention of this complication if at all possible. Most authors splint only the DIP joint in extension or slight hyperextension and allow full active motion of the proximal joints. Blue[45] states that he has found immobilization of the PIP joint for these injuries clinically unnecessary.

A clinical study comparing the methods of immobilization would be most interesting as the method allowing some tension on the repair, i.e., immobilization of the DIP joint only allows some tendon "function" during the repair process, while the other methods eliminate or reduce any tension on the repair.

The methods of immobilizing the DIP joint only are certainly functionally less restricting to the patient, which is an important consideration, since the immobilization period is so lengthy. With a splint and/or K-wire that effectively immobilizes the joint with no danger of slippage, most patients can continue working in some capacity.

Mobilization Period.   After immobilization for 6 to 8 weeks, free active range of motion is begun. The major problems encountered are most commonly associated with a recurrence of the deformity due to attenuation of the repaired tendon. If the tendon has healed with a scar that is too long or if the inititation of motion causes attenuation of the tendon unit, full active extension of the distal joint will not be possible. In these cases, splinting to maintain distal joint extension should be resumed, in order to encourage remodelling of the repaired tendon scar in a shortened, more favorable position. During this period, the splint should be removed for a few minutes at least three times a day to allow active flexion exercise. Despite the attempt to establish a shortened tendon with extension splinting, active flexion should be begun by the eighth week to begin counteracting the joint changes caused by immobilization. Functionally, it is sometimes more important to compromise extension somewhat in order to regain full flexion. Care must be taken, however, to prevent recurrence of a mallet finger, which will potentially lead to the imbalance causing PIP joint hyperextension.

After extended periods of immobilization with the distal joint in extension, some younger patients are immediately able to fully flex the DIP joint upon removal of the splint. Very often, these patients develop a recurrent mallet finger. These patients may require longer periods of extension immobilization and a more guarded active flexion program, perhaps utilizing a dynamic extension splint to assist distal joint extension. Conversely, it may take an older patient many months to regain flexion, due to fibrosis around the joint. Passive flexion therapeutic measures may be needed, using flexion splinting and joint mobilization to regain functional active flexion.

FLEXOR TENDON MANAGEMENT

General Considerations

Despite advances in surgical technique, management of a newly repaired flexor tendon still presents a challenge! Although numerous variations in postoperative managements are practiced, all have the common goal of preventing the formation of restricting adhesions.[16,17,25,56,57] The authors have come to expect different results with injuries to different anatomic locations of the flexor tendons.[18] Innovations in management focus primarily on flexor tendons within the digital sheath, because they frequently have such poor functional results. The problem is a biological one and not a technical one, as the required differential remodeling of a single scar is not yet within our control.[12,52]

The issue of when to start motion following repair remains unsettled. Advances in flexor tendon management center around the initiation of "early controlled mobilization." To the student unfamiliar with flexor tendon management, this term can be misleading. This does not entail *active* motion of the newly repaired tendon, and the majority of surgeons still advocate *no* unprotected active motion before 3 weeks after repair.[16,17,30,36,39,52,57] The development of different techniques of tendon suture prompted a few authors to initiate early active motion.[56,58] These sutures were reported to have greater tensile strength and less gap formation when placed under tension, thus allowing for the stress of active motion. Nevertheless, early active motion has not gained wide acceptance, and the most widely used and reported managements today are (1) classic 3-week immobilization period, (2) controlled passive motion, and (3) early controlled mobilization with active extension.

The choice of a postoperative management will be influenced by the individual surgeon's belief as to how a tendon heals. He/she may choose one management method and never waver from it. On the other hand, the surgeon and the therapist together may consider each case individually, perhaps choosing one appropriate method for that patient or take bits and pieces from several methods, creating a truly trailor-made program. No matter the choice of management, it will be aimed at influencing the physical properties of scar tissues. The goals of any method of management include (1) adequate tensile strength of the anastomosis, (2) the prevention of adhesions which limit tendon gliding, (3) a functional range of joint motion, and (4) preservation of function of the uninvolved digits.

The therapist responsible for managing a tendon repair must go beyond what surgeons report in the literature. Even if a therapist uses the prescribed protocol of either Peacock,[36] Duran and Houser,[16] or Kleinert,[18,39] at some point he/she may wish to tailor the treatment with the intelligent and careful use of the other modalities and procedures in physical medicine.

Stages of scar maturation must be considered, as well as soft tissue reaction to the procedure. Although the authors have no direct evidence that any of their treatment methods can favorably influence scar remodeling, clinically they have witnessed the effectiveness of the timely and judicious use of the application of stress. The research study of Arem and Madden[37] supports this concept. They created a model in the rat to test the hypothesis that properly timed application of stress could affect scar remodeling. Their results offer exciting implications for the field of tendon management. They found that scar subjected to stress at 3 weeks was markedly elongated. Also of significance was the finding that mature scar of fourteen weeks subjected to stress was virtually indistinguishable from the unstressed controlled scar.

Active exercise subjects a tendon to stress, and gentle PIP flexion with the MP blocked in extension is commonly initiated at 3 to 3½ weeks. Graded active exercise is often enough to produce a functional degree of tendon excursion. However, if lack of tendon excursion remains a problem, additional procedures may favorably influence the return of active motion. At 8 weeks, scar maturation between the tendon ends is sufficiently strong to withstand loading,[36] and the circumferential scar about the tendon still, theoretically, has the potential to elongate. At this point, electrical muscle stimulation may be utilized to facilitate tendon excursion as well as to stress the restricting adhesions. The combined application of heat and stretch produces significant elongation of rat tail tendon,[59] and may have a favorable influence on the elongation of tendon adhesions. Ultrasound is known to selectively heat tissues high in collagen content,[60] and may be useful in raising the temperature of scar tissue within the therapeutic range. This rise in temperature, combined with active tendon gliding exercises may result in residual elongation of the restricting scar.[59] Extreme caution is necessary when using ultrasound on a recently repaired tendon, as its effects on tendon healing are not fully understood. Although there are reports of its stimulating potential in tissue regeneration in open wounds,[60] ultrasound utilized on freshly healing tendon repairs in rabbits for a 6-week period was found to adversely affect healing. However, once cross-linking has been established, and loading has been initiated after 7 to 8 weeks, ultrasound may be used safely and effectively, in our opinion.[61]

Any postoperative management program is geared toward the gradual gain in tendon excursion, as a result of slowly developing changes in the physical characteristics of the scar. Attempting to "break adhesions" has no place in tendon management,[34] and only serves to set off an inflammatory reaction that ultimately will result in yet more scar formation. The therapist, then, must carefully grade the amount of vigorous active motion in order to avoid this undesirable consequence.

Management by Immobilization

The classic 3 weeks of postoperative immobilization is not new; however, it continues to be used today and is, in our opinion, still the management of choice for unreliable patients.

The wrist is immobilized in a neutral position, and tension across the anastomosis is relieved by flexing the MPs and PIPs.[36] Rather than leaving the dressing undisturbed for the entire immobilization period, in patients over 35 years of age it is recommended to put the joints through passive range of motion every 7 to 10 days. Older patients are almost certain to have problems with joint stiffness, and it is far easier to prevent joint contractures than to correct them once they have occurred. With the wrist and MP joints held in flexion, the PIP joint is passively moved through its complete range. An alternative to this is to simply immobilize the patient for the full 3 weeks with the wrist in slight flexion, the MCPs in flexion, and the PIPs and DIPs in neutral. Passive motion to avoid a PIP flexion contracture then becomes unnecessary. Protective splinting is usually discontinued after 3 to 4 weeks, unless the patient's "vigorous" lifestyle necessitates protection for longer. Once the splint is removed at 3 weeks, passive flexion and gentle active flexion are initiated at the same time. Blocking exercises for the MCP first and the PIP later, passive stretch into extension, and dynamic/static extension splints can all gradually be added along a time line, as the biology of tendon repair allows and as the patient demonstrates need. Most improvement usually occurs within the first 12 weeks, although it is not uncommon for improvement to continue beyond this point.

Management by Controlled Passive Motion

The concept of controlled passive motion is not entirely new, although it has recently increased in popularity. Young and Harmon[57] reported a technique of passive motion in 1960, and introduced the concept of nail suture and elastic traction. In their report, the patient passively extended the digit against the rubber band, and upon release the band passively brought it back to the partially flexed resting posture. The most widely used method of controlled passive motion is that described by Duran and Houser.[16] It is based on the premise that a passive extension movement resulting in 3 to 5 mm of tendon excursion will help to prevent adherence of the repaired flexor tendon in Zones II and III. The effects of controlled passive motion on tendon repair has been studied experimentally using canine tendons.[35,62] Passive motion was instituted immediately in one group and at 3 weeks in another. Strength properties in the early, protected mobilized tendons (represented by the ultimate failure load and linear slope) were significantly better, as was tendon excursion with *passive* motion.

Controlled passive motion, as used clinically, either begins immediately[16] or between 2 to 5 days postoperatively.[63] Duran and Houser provide a very exacting protocol, which calls for determination, at the time of surgery, of the degrees of PIP and DIP passive extension required to see the anastomosis glide 3 to 5 mm. The wrist is immobilized in 20 to 30° of flexion, and the digits are held in a balanced position. The involved digit is secured in flexion by its attachment to a rubber band connected to the volar aspect of the wrist. A modified version[63] utilizes a dorsal protective splint immobilizing the wrist and digits, without the use of rubber band traction.

Twice a day, passive motion of the involved digit's PIP and DIP is carried out within the pre-determined range[16] or within the confines of the dorsal splint.[63] The DIP is passively extended to separate the repair sites of the FDP and FDS. The PIP is passively extended to separate both tendons from the surrounding fixed structures of the fibro-osseous tunnel. This routine is carried out for 4½ weeks.

It is interesting to note here the difference in the timing of initiation of active motion. After management by immobilization, active motion is allowed at 3 weeks, in contrast to 4½ weeks in the controlled passive motion technique. The delay in initiation of active motion in this case is based on the premise that a tendon managed in this way has healed mostly through intrinsic mechanisms. Therefore, because peripheral adhesions did not contribute to its healing process, the anastomosis may be weaker and requires protection from active motion for longer than do immobilized tendons.

At 4½ weeks, the rubber band traction is transferred to a wrist cuff, and gentle active flexion and extension exercises are allowed. At 5½ weeks, all protective splinting is discontinued, and active exercises are gradually increased.[16] This management technique requires very careful patient selection—the patient is not only required to assume responsibility for his twice daily passive extension exercises, but he/she must be willing to return to the clinic for frequent follow-up visits.

Management by Early Controlled Mobilization

Kleinert's method of immediate, controlled mobilization is perhaps the most widely used, and has popularized the rubber band traction introduced by Young and Harmon in 1960.[57] It was developed for the problematic flexors in Zone II, although recently the utilization of this method is described in the management of injuries in the other zones as well.[18]

The hand is immobilized with either an immediate postoperative dorsal plaster splint or a splint fabricated from one of the commercially available thermoplastic materials. As Kleinert describes it,[39] this splint extends from the proximal forearm to beyond the fingertips, and includes all the fingers. A modification of this original splint uses a dorsal extension for the repaired digit only.[17] The wrist is kept in 30 to 45° of flexion, the MP joints slightly flexed from 0 to 20° and the IPs may be allowed to fully extend (Fig. 2-9). A rubber band connects the nail loop with a safety pin secured at the wrist, so that the tension on the rubber band keeps the finger in flexion. One of the most common complications of this method is a PIP flexion contracture. This can be avoided by careful monitoring of the tension of the rubber band; it should never be strong enough to impede full PIP and DIP extension to the limits established by the splint. Fabricating the splint so that the PIP is at 0° extension, and assurance that the patient is able to extend fully so that the dorsum of the finger contacts the splint should prevent this complication from occurring. Three days after repair, active extension within the confines of the splint is begun. The patient is taught to relax and allow the recoil of the rubber band to passively flex the digit to its previous flexed posture. This is repeated six times, for a total of four to six times per day.

Kleinert reports that EMG studies confirm that during active digital extension, the digital flexors are in a state of relaxation.[18,39] Active flexion is not begun until 24 days after repair. Again, it is interesting to note the difference in the time frame for active

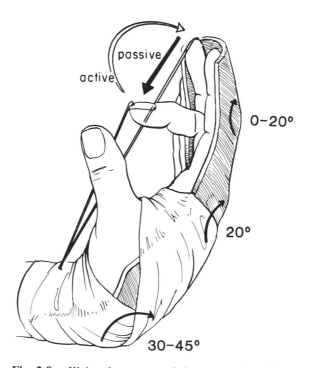

Fig. 2-9. Kleinert's recommended postoperative splint.

flexion. The one common bond among all managements is that no active flexion is allowed before 3 weeks of healing has taken place. If only the FDP was repaired, rubber band traction attached to a wrist cuff is continued for another 2 weeks. As previously described with the tendon's blood supply, the vinculum longus to the FDP in Zone II is a continuation of the vinculum brevis to the FDS. So without the FDS, the blood supply to the repaired profundus is compromised, which likely results in delayed healing. Power flexion activities are avoided until 8 weeks postoperatively, as in all types of management.[16,36,39]

Research into the mechanisms of tendon repair stimulated the development of new management techniques to incorporate our increasing knowledge. The reported success in achieving excellent or good results with both of the controlled mobilization techniques[17,18,63] seems to reflect a better understanding and utilization of tendon healing principles in postoperative management. The key term here is "controlled mobilization." Peacock points out that the amount of early motion is not extensive enough to prevent revascularization.[36] That the extent of motion is small is supported by Duran and Houser's measurement of 3 to 5 mm and other investigators' measurement of approximately 1 mm of excursion for 10 degress of joint flexion in Zone II.[26] Paratendinous tissues may still provide the reparative cells, but they do so through favorable adhesions that allow a longitudinal excursion of the tendon.

The ultimate postoperative flexor tendon management has yet to be found. In fact, the pursuit of one generally accepted management technique seems unrealistic, even impossible. A choice of management should be based on several factors—the nature and extent of the injury, the anticipated extrinsic and intrinsic response to injury, the patient's age, occupation, environmental and psychological factors—none of which will ever be exactly the same in any two patients. How, then, can we expect a predetermined treatment protocol to meet the needs of each individual? It is the opinion of these authors that perhaps the most significant "advance in tendon management" is really the combined ability of the therapist and the surgeon to compile bits and pieces from the varying management philosophies in order to tailor an individually appropriate program for each patient.

CONCLUSIONS

Research into the mechanisms of tendon healing has clearly helped to change our philosophy of flexor and extensor tendon management. The desire to prevent or control adhesion formation has been a potent stimulus in the development of these changes. A tendon may "choose" to heal in three ways, and an understanding of the clinical factors that influence this choice forms the basis for the management techniques discussed in this chapter.

Technical advances in tendon surgery have already helped to diminish the formation of adhesions in response to the trauma of surgery. The future holds exciting possibilites in the pharmacological control of scar. Further advances are also dependent upon progress in postoperative management. This challenges us to contribute to the field by investigating the effects of our treatment methods, keeping accurate records, and continuing to ask questions so that new ideas can be developed into clinical advancements.

REFERENCES

1. Mason M, Allen H: The rate of healing tendons. Ann Surg 113:424, 1941
2. Brockis JG: The blood supply of the flexor and extensor tendons of the fingers in man. J Bone Joint Surg 35-B: Feb. 1953
3. Caplan H, Hunter J, Merklin R: Intrinsic vascularization of flexor tendons. p. 48. In AAOS Symposium on Tendon Surgery in the Hand. CV Mosby Co, St Louis, 1975
4. Edwards D: The blood supply and lymphatic drainage of tendons. J Anat 80: 147, 1946
5. Lundborg G, Myrhage R, Ryedvik B: The vascularization of human flexor tendons within the digital synovial sheath region structural and functional aspects. J Hand Surg 2:417, 1977
6. Peacock EE: A study of the circulation in normal tendons and healing grafts. Ann Surg 149:415, 1959
7. Smith J: Blood supply of tendons. Am J Surg 109:272, 1978
8. Bergljung L: Vascular reactions in tendon healing. Angiology 21: 375, 1970
9. Mathews JP: Vascular changes in flexor tendons after injury and repair: An experimental study. Injury 8:227, 1979
10. Furlow LT: The role of tendon tissues in tendon healing. Plast Reconstr Surg 57:39, 1976
11. Lindsay WK, Thomson HG: Digital flexor tendons: An experimental study. Br J Plast Surg 12:289, 1960
12. Peacock EE: Biological principles in the healing of long tendons. Surg Clin North Am 45:2, 461, 1965
13. Potenza A: Tendon healing within the flexor digital sheath in the dog. J Bone Joint Surg 44A:49, 1962
14. Colville J, Callison JR, White, WL: Role of Mesotenon in Tendon Blood Supply. Plast Reconstr Surg 43: 53, 1969
15. Ochiai N, Matsui T, Miyaji N et al: Vascular anatomy of flexor tendons. I Vincular system and blood supply of the profundus tendon in the digital sheath. J Hand Surg 4:321, 1979
16. Duran RJ, Houser RG: Controlled passive motion following flexor tendon repair in zones II and II. p. 105. In AAOS Symposium on Tendon Surgery in the Hand. C V Mosby Co, St. Louis, 1975
17. Earley MJ, Milward TM: The primary repair of digital flexor tendons. Br J Plast Surg 35:133, 1982
18. Kleinert HE, Schepel S, Gill T: Flexor tendon injuries. Surg Clin North Am 61:267, 1981
19. Doyle J, Blythe W: The flexor tendon sheath and pulleys: Anatomy and reconstruction. p. 81. In AAOS Symposium on Tendon Surgery in the Hand. CV Mosby Co, St Louis, 1975
20. Lundborg G, Myrhage R: The vascularization and structure of the human digital tendon sheath as related to flexor tendon function. Scand J Plast Reconstr Surg 11:195, 1977
21. McDowell C, Synder D: Tendon healing: An experimental model in the dog. J Hand Surg 2:122, 1977
22. Potenza A: Critical evaluation of flexor-tendon healing and adhesion formation within artificial digital sheaths. J Bone Joint Surg 45A: 1217, 1963
23. Lundborg G, Rank F: Experimental intrinsic healing of flexor tendons based upon synovial fluid nutrition, J Hand Surg 3:21, 1978
24. Manske P, Birdwell K, Lesker P: Nutrient pathways to flexor tendons of chickens using tritiated proline. J Hand Surg 3:352, 1978
25. Becker H, Graham M, Cohen IK, Diegelmann R: Intrinsic tendon cell proliferation in tissue culture. J Hand Surg 66:616, 1981
26. McGrouther DA, Ahmed MR: Flexor tendon excursions in "No-Man's Land." Hand 13:129, 1981
27. Lundborg G, Rank F: Experimental studies on cellular mechanisms involved in healing of animal and human flexor tendon in synovial environment. Hand 12:3, 1980

28. Manske P, Gelberman R et al: Intrinsic flexor tendon repair. J Bone Joint Surg 66A:385, 1984
29. Boyes J: Discussion section of Symposium on the Hand, Elliott, Vol. 3, 1971
30. Ketchum L: Primary tendon healing: A review. J Hand Surg 2(6):428, 1977
31. Mason M, Shearon C: The process of tendon repair. Arch Surg 25:615, 1932
32. Matthews P, Richards H: Factors in the adherence of flexor tendons after repair. J Bone Joint Surg 58B: 230, 1976
33. Potenza A: Effect of associated trauma on healing of divided tendons. J Trauma 2:173, 1962
34. Weiner L, Peacock E: Biologic principles affecting repair of flexor tendons. Adv Surg 5:145, 1971
35. Woo S, Gelberman R et al: The importance of controlled passive mobilization in flexor tendon healing. Acta Orthop Scand 52: 615, 1981
36. Peacock E, Madden J, Trier W: Postoperative recovery of flexor tendon function. Am J Surg 122:686, 1971
37. Arem A, Madden J: Effects of stress on healing wounds: I. Intermittent noncyclical tension. J Surg Res 20: 93, 1976
38. Dargan EL: Management of extensor tendon injuries of the hand. Surg Gynecol Obstet 128: 1269, 1969
39. Kleinert HE, Kutz JE, Cohen M: Primary repair of the zone 2 flexor tendon lacerations. p. 91. In AAOS Symposium on Tendon Surgery in the Hand. CV Mosby Co, St. Louis, 1975
40. Elliot RA: Injuries to the extensor mechanism of the hand. Orthop Clin North Am 1(2):335, 1970
41. Eiken O, Hagberg L, Lundborg G: Evolving biologic concepts as applied to tendon surgery. Clin Plast Surg 8(1):1, 1981
42. Zbrodowski A, Gajisin S, Grodeki J: Vascularization and anatomical model of the mesotendons of the extensor digitorum and extensor indicis muscles. J Anat 130(4):697, 1980
43. Nemethi E: Extensor tendons in the industrially injured hand. Indust M & S 113, March 1956
44. Sakellarides HT: The extensor tendon injuries and the treatment. RI Med J 307 Aug. 1978
45. Blue A, Spira M, Hardy S: Repair of extensor tendon injuries of the hand. Am J Surg 132, 128, 1976
46. Zbrodowski A: Anatomic model of the ligamentous apparatus of the tendons of the extensor digitorum muscle of the hand in man. Folia Morphol 32: 381, 1973
47. Kaplan EB: Anatomy, injuries and treatment of the extensor apparatus of the hand and digits. Clin Orthop 13:24, 1959
48. Stuart D: Duration of splinting after repair of extensor tendons in the hand. J Bone Joint Surg 47B: 1; 70, 1965
49. Donatelli R, Owens-Burkhart H: Effects of immobilization on the extensibility of periarticular connective tissue. J Orthop Sports PT 3:2, 67, 1981
50. Lavigne A: Imobilization induced stiffness of monkey knee joints and posterior capsule. Perspectives in Biomedical Engineering. Univ Park Press, Baltimore, June 1972
51. Rosenthal E: The Extensor Tendons. p. 197. In Hunter JM, Schneider LH, Mackin EJ: Rehabilitation of the Hand. CV Mosby Co, St Louis; 1978
52. Merritt WH: Complications of hand surgery and trauma. In Greenfield LJ (ed): Complications in Surgery and Trauma. JB Lippincott, Philadelphia, 1984
53. Tubiana R, Valentin P: The physiology of extension of the fingers. Surg Clin North Am 44(4):907, 1964
54. Boyes Joseph H: Bunnell's Surgery of the Hand. 5th Ed. JB Lippincott Co, Philadelphia, p. 13, 1970
55. Harris C, Rutledge G: The functional anatomy of the extensor mechanism of the finger. J Bone Joint Surg 54-A 4: 713, 1972

56. Kessler I, Nissim F: Primary repair without immobilization of flexor tendon division within the digital sheath. Acta Orthop Scand 40:587, 1969

57. Young R, Harmon J: Repair of tendon injuries of the hand. Ann Surg 151:562, 1960

58. Becker H, Orak F, Duponselle E: Early active motion following a beveled technique of flexor tendon repair: Report on fifty cases. J Hand Surg 4(5):454, 1979

59. Warren CG, Lehman JF, Koblanski J: Elongation of rat tail tendon: Effect of load and temperature. Arch Phys Med Rehabil 52:465, 1971

60. Dyson M, Suckling J: Stimulation of tissue repair by ultrasound: A survey of the mechanisms involved. Physiotherapy 64:105, 1978

61. Roberts M et al: The effect of ultrasound on flexor tendon repairs in rabbits. Hand 14:17, 1982

62. Gelberman RH et al: Effects of early intermittent passive mobilization on healing canine flextor tendons. J Hand Surg 7(2):170, 1982

63. Strickland JW, Glogovac SV: Digital function following flexor tendon repair in zone II: a comparison of immobilization and controlled passive motion techniques. J Hand Surg 5:537, 1980

3 | Sensibility Measurement and Management

Christine A. Moran
Anne D. Callahan

Sensory testing has long been viewed as a necessary yet time consuming aspect of peripheral nerve rehabilitation. Part of the difficulty stems from the vast number of tests available and the extensiveness of the hand area to be tested. Yet important information about the progression of nerve compression and nerve regeneration can be obtained from careful, regular testing.

As will be discussed in the section on historical perspective, sensory testing is founded in neurological testing. Neurologists use the modality tests to ascertain central nervous system integrity and spinal tract continuity. These tests (pinprick, touch, hot/cold, vibration) assess those areas, but do not completely assess the status of the peripheral nervous system.

This chapter will discuss the development and growth of sensory tests, parameters of sensory testing, the rationale of sensory re-education, and sensory training itself. This aspect of hand rehabilitation is still controversial and will require additional laboratory and clinical research. The reader is encouraged to remember that the following are current guidelines.

Terms first need to be defined. Is it sensation or sensibility? *Sensation* is defined as the physiological discharge of skin mechanoreceptors, nociceptors, and thermoreceptors, due to the application of a stimulus and the subsequent activation of a volley of afferent neural impulses, and measurable via electrodiagnostic methods.[1,2] *Sensibility*, on the other hand, is the cortical interpretation and appreciation of an external stimulus applied to the skin, and is measured with sensory tests.[2-4] Therefore, sensation is the physiological mechanism, and sensibility is the ability of the patient to interpret the stimuli.

The second set of terms needing definition are functional sensibility and academic sensibility. Functional sensibility indicates the patient's ability to use his recovered sensibility for fine prehension, daily activities, and work, while academic sensibility describes the presence or absence of that specific parameter of sensation tested.[2,5] Tests that give functional information are two-point discrimination (static and moving), the pick-up test, and braille designs, while tests like light touch, and pinprick describe academic sensibility.[5]

HISTORICAL PERSPECTIVE

In the 1880s, Von Frey and Blix devised the first tests for measuring sensations of warmth, cold, pain, and touch.[6,7] These tests were developed as peripheral measurements to document lesions in the central nervous system in their patients.

Weber, in 1845, reported a series of sensory studies in which he described a Two-Point Discrimination (2PD) test.[8] Using a caliper as the testing instrument, he identified the variation in normal body part sensitivity and devised mappings of two-point sensitivity. Although little was known about the structure and function of skin receptors, Weber suggested that touch sensitivity varied throughout the body due to receptor density. Additionally, he postulated that a moving object is perceived more easily than a static object placed on the skin surface, and that sensation is learned. Later works have substantiated and confirmed Weber's early findings.[9-16]

Von Frey devised another test for measuring touch by creating a series of hand-held instruments from wooden rods with an individual hair glued to the end.[7] Each rod carried a successively larger diameter hair, which could be touched to the skin, and these became known as Von Frey hairs. Von Frey proposed that this test measured the threshold for light touch, and identified the location of "touch spots."[6,17,18]

The testing of sensation was studied largely by neurophysiologists, psychologists, and neurologists until World War I. During World War I and II, many American and European surgeons were treating peripheral nerve war injuries, and became concerned about the sensitivity and reliability of the sensory measurement tests available to them to accurately evaluate the patient's recovering sensation.[15,16,18,19] As a result, many tests were developed, as outlined in Table 3-1. As the tests were developed, they were used separately or in groups.

Starting in the late 1950s, comparative studies of sensory tests were conducted. Seddon reported the usefulness of combining academic and functional tests for measuring the patient's sensory progress when he outlined an evaluation series of 2PD, light touch, and the coin test.[18] Moberg observed in 1958 a non-statistical positive relationship of nerve recovery to 2PD, grip, the pickup test, and sudomotor recovery in seven nerve repair patients.[16]

Weinstein, in a series of studies, updated and standardized the Von Frey test and renamed the test the Semmes-Weinstein monofilament test.[4,20,21] Weinstein's laboratory studies confirmed the body part sensitivity tests of Weber and provided detailed light touch mappings of normal males and females. During this period, Von Prince

Table 3-1. Clinical Sensory Tests 1800–1980

Test	Author	Date
Light touch	Blix, Von Frey	1830–1840
Temperature	Blix, Von Frey	1830–1840
Pinprick	Blix, Von Frey	1830–1840
Vibration	Blix, Von Frey	1830–1840
Two-point discrimination	Weber	1845
Von Frey hairs	Von Frey	1895
Tinel's sign	Tinel	1915
Coin test	Riddoch, Seddon	1940–1956
Ninhydrine sweat test	Guttman	1940
Pressure test	Nafe	1941
V-Test	Mackworth	1953
Von Frey stimulator	Weddell	1955
Ninhydrine sweat test	Moberg	1954
Pickup test	Moberg	1958
Renfrew ridge	Renfrew	1960
Semmes-Weinstein monofilaments	Weinstein, Semmes	1962
Size discrimination test	Vierck, Jones	1969
Modified pressure test	Jaminson	1972
Finger wrinkling test	O'Riain	1973
Depth/spatial instruments	Carlson	1974
Automated pressure, thermal vibration tests	Dyck	1976
Optacon	Craig	1976
Light touch filament	Naafs, Dagne	1977
Finger wrinkling test	Phelps	1977
Moving two-point discrimination	Dellon	1978
Braille designs	Millesi	1978
Tactile/thermal instrumentation	De Michelis	1979
Prototype pressure anesthesiometer	Kanatani	1979
Automated pressure test	Looft, Williams	1979
Ridge device/sensiometer	Poppen	1979
Vibration discrimination	Dellon	1980
Edshage arrow test	Edshage	1980

From Moran CA: Comparison of sensory testing methods using carpal tunnel syndrome patients. Unpublished Master's Thesis, Medical College of Virginia, 1981.

began using the monofilaments for clinical testing of over 100 peripheral nerve-injured patients, and devised a table of recovering sensory values different from Weinstein.[22,23] Over 4,000 tests were conducted by Von Prince and Werner using the 2PD test and the Semmes-Weinstein test.[23,24] Their clinical findings demonstrated the necessity of using both the Semmes-Weinstein test for light touch measurement and the 2PD test for spatial measurement.

Onne studied the reliability of several sensory tests on 45 peripheral nerve patients.[25] He compared the four modalities of pain, cold, warmth, and touch (pinprick, Von Frey touch test) to tactile gnosis (2PD, coin test, pick-up test, localization test) and to sudomotor function (ninhydrine sweat test). By plotting test values, he identified a close relationship between the patient's age and 2PD test, and that 2PD decreased with age. He concluded from his results that both 2PD and the pick-up test were reliable indicators of functional sensibility, but that the touch test and the ninhydrine test were not. Flynn and Flynn also compared the ninhydrine test to the pick-up test, the 2PD test, and the coin test in a long-term study of peripheral nerve-injured patients, and found that the ninhydrine test was the most objective indicator of recovering sensation.[26]

Renfrew compared the sensitivity of his test for spatial and depth sense, the Renfrew ridge, to the 2PD test and an object identification test for measuring sensibility, in 10 normal subjects and later in 40 patients with central nervous system lesions.[14,27] He found the test ridge to be more sensitive, by reporting that depth sense threshold was raised in 36 hands of 28 patients tested who had normal 2PD. He found the ridge test easy to use, and pointed out that the ridge test measured depth-spatial perception not measured by the other instruments. Porter designed functional block tests of letters, compared these tests to other sensory tests such as 2PD and pick-up tests, and found the block tests more sensitive and easier to administer, when compared to the other tests.[28] Edshage has reported preliminary results of an arrow block test, but has noted that further studies are needed.[29]

In 1972, Dellon, Curtis, and Edgerton reported a series of sensory tests that would detect recovery of the slow-adapting and quickly adapting receptor-fiber system.[30] The tests were light stroking, constant touch, vibration at 30 c/s and 256 c/s, pinprick, and 2PD. They reported accurate documentation of recovery with these tests using 12 peripheral nerve-injured patients.

Dellon described a moving version of the 2PD test which he felt would measure the early recovery of quickly adapting receptors.[12,31] In his studies, he documented recovery of moving 2PD before static 2PD in both peripheral nerve repair and compression patients by plotting test values for static and moving 2PD. He noted that the improvements in moving 2PD coincided with improvements in the patients' functional abilities more frequently than did 2PD. In 1980, he introduced a new version of the vibration test for reportedly monitoring the early recovery of nerve fibers that mediate quickly adapting sensory stimuli.[32] In this 2-year study of 101 patients, he noted that altered vibratory sense was observed in more patients more frequently and was recovered from earlier than the other sensations. Reviewing the study's sample of CTS patients, Dellon noted that 72 percent of the patients had altered vibratory sense, while 50 percent had altered moving 2PD and static 2PD, 70 percent had positive Phalen's test, and 63 percent had prolonged nerve conduction studies.

Poppen published a long-term study of 49 digital nerve and 14 peripheral nerve patients using the Sensiometer, a modification of the Renfrew ridge, to evaluate the recovery of moving tactile gnosis.[10] Graphically comparing the Semmes-Weinstein monofilament, the 2PD, and the Sensiometer, he reported that the Sensiometer detected more changes in tactile gnosis within the range of 8-12 mm in 2PD.

Other tests were designed or adapted from 1960 to 1980, though comparative studies were not made. Phelps and Walker[33] and O'Riain[34] independently described the finger wrinkling test as a visible measure of recovering sudomotor function and thus sensory function, based on Moberg's and Guttman's earlier works of simultaneous sudomotor and nerve recovery.[16,35] Vierck and Jones introduced a size discrimination test using solid plastic cylinders of varying diameters for measuring spatial discrimination not detected by the 2PD test and for monitoring functional recovery of sensation.[36] Modifications of the Semmes-Weinstein test[37] and the Renfrew ridge[38] were also introduced. Using the Optacon,[39] originally designed for Braille readers and recently tested for sensitivity and reliability, Arezzo and Schaumberg tested 100 normal subjects and

24 diabetics.[40] They reported that the Optacon detected sensory changes not previously measured in the diabetic group and also had the ability to detect threshold differences in normal subjects of varying ages. These researchers hope to utilize the Optacon clinically, as the testing requires only 5 minutes and, thus far, studies demonstrate sensitivity and reliability.

Other researchers also sought more reliable measures using automation. Dyck reported that the clinical tests available contained too many uncontrolled variables.[41] Almost all instruments were handheld, stimulus probes were of different diameters, skin indentation was not controlled, and data analysis was subjective.[41-43] As an alternative, an automated systems instrument unit, designed at the Mayo Clinics, eliminated all of the aforementioned variables. The testing unit demonstrates a sophisticated sensitivity by incorporating a forced choice technique to reduce response bias.[39] However, all of Dyck's studies to date have been conducted on the non-glabrous skin of patients with central and peripheral nervous system lesions. Also concerned with the inadequacies of the handheld instruments, DeMichelis et al and Looft and Williams introduced automated instrumentation for quantifying sensory changes.[44,45] Levin and his colleagues, rather than introduce another instrument, conducted an engineering analysis of the Semmes-Weinstein instrument.[46] They cited the following problems of the instrument. First, the instrument should be calibrated in stress units rather than force units only. Second, the lack of uniformity of the probe tips alters force application. Third, the improper gluing of the filament into the probe handle causes the filament to buckle at a lower force during application. Last, the elastic modulus of the filament changes with variations in temperature and humidity.

The need for sensitive and reliable tests in measuring nontraumatic sensory loss such as occurs in diabetes also leads to more reported studies. These studies also contribute to the continued investigation of sensory testing.[47-49] Chockinov and colleagues found, in comparing 53 juvenile diabetics to their relatives (n = 51), a significantly higher threshold of 2PD in the diabetic group when sensory nerve conduction, motor nerve conduction, 2PD, and touch tests were compared ($P<.001$).[47] Comparing diabetics and non-diabetics, Gregarson (1968) found changes in vibratory perception that coincided with duration of disease and the subject's age ($P<.05$).[48] Heinrich and Moorhouse used vibration, Von Frey test, and 2PD for comparison of sensory levels in 10 blind subjects, 10 blind diabetic subjects, and 10 sighted subjects.[49] Their findings showed that there was no significant difference between the sighted and blind subjects ($P<.9$, $P<.5$, $P<.4$) with these tests. However, all thresholds for the blind diabetic subjects were significantly higher for all tests ($P<.01$, $P<.01$, $P<.001$), when compared to the threshold values of the sighted and blind subjects.

Lundborg also rejected findings of non-traumatic sensory loss via experimentally induced median nerve compression at the carpal tunnel.[50] In 16 volunteer subjects, varying pressures were administered for different lengths of time. Their results showed that sensory conduction block occurred much earlier than the motor conduction block, and 2PD remained within normal limits until the last stage of sensory fiber conduction. A later study demonstrated similar findings, with abnormal vibrometer and Semmes-Weinstein monofilament readings much earlier than abnormal 2PD readings.[51] This author also identified the same pattern of sensory test abnormalities in a group of patients with carpal tunnel syndrome.[52] Consistently in the study, the Semmes-Weinstein monofilaments detected sensory changes when 2PD was recorded within normal limits.

To place all this historical information into perspective, let us briefly review the theories of sensation. Each theory was developed based on the understanding of sensation and sensibility at that time. They also help to better understand the complex nature of sensation and sensibility and, therefore, testing and retraining.

The Specificity Theory (1895)

Von Frey presented this revolutionary theory based on Muller's Specific Energy Theory described in 1838.[7,53] Muller's Theory stated that one stimulus to one afferent nerve produced only one sensation, and yet if the same stimulus was applied to another nerve, a different sensation would be produced. Von Frey expanded this theory and produced a new sense of order and direction in sensory research.[54] His theory states that each skin receptor is specialized and responds to only one stimulus. Each receptor is directly connected to a specific center in the cortex via certain afferent fibers.[7,55] Von Frey indentified four modalities of sensation (pain, pressure, warm, cold) and their corresponding skin receptors (free nerve endings, Meissner's corpuscles, Ruffini cylinders, Krause bulbs), and observed that each receptor could be detected within the touch spots earlier described by Blix.[6]

The Theory of Head (1905)

Head's theory developed from his observations of documented nerve recovery from a transected sensory nerve in his arm.[56] He outlined three defined areas of specific sensation, which he labeled anesthesia, protopathic sensation, and epicritic sensation. He defined protopathic sensation as gross temperature and pain, whereas epicritic sensation pertained to light touch, tactile localization, and fine temperature changes. From these observations, Head devised a system of duality for nerve regeneration, where protopathic sensation or general sensation recovered first and more quickly than the epicritic sensation or specific sensation. Thus, during nerve regeneration, pain and temperature recovered first, followed by touch, tactile localization, and fine changes in temperature.

Pattern Theory (1927)

Nafe, drawing from Adrian's work on single fiber recordings, developed the pattern theory, which states that all perception of sensation is derived by patterns of neural discharge and not from specialized receptors.[6,57] The patterns are derived from the variations of impulse trains, the duration of impulse discharge, the area of skin stimulated, and the number of fibers activated. The specialization of sensation was not found at the receptor level but rather at the cortical level. Nafe conducted a series of studies to verify his theory, using copper stimulus probes of different diameters and temperatures. The subjects in these studies reported several sensations rather than one sensation, according to Nafe.

Many authors have applauded and criticized these theories as explanations of sensation. Though Von Frey's theory was revolutionary, specific areas of the theory were empirically derived. First, Goldscheider objected to the inclusion of pain as a modality of sensation.[55] Secondly, the theory implied a specific one to one relationship between the psychological sensory component and the physical stimulus.[53] Thus, the theory fails to account for a wide range of sensory experiences.[6,56] Sherrington observed that the receptor is only an apparatus that makes the afferent nerve more receptive to the physical stimulus, rather than serving as the basis of sensation.[57] Melzack and Wall, while examining Von Frey's three assumptions, noted that his physiological assumption is the theory's strength and the reason for its survival as a theory. Mountcastle confirms the importance of Von Frey's receptor identification by citing the scientific acknowledgement of receptor specificity to a greater degree than Von Frey originally outlined.[3]

Von Frey, in a conference address, reaffirmed the plausibility of his theory, in which he emphasized the ease in detecting receptors within specific touch spots.[7] He observed that the continuous perception of sensation is due to physical and physiological irradiation of the stimulus rather than to many different receptors closely spaced. Von Frey also refuted Head's theory by explaining the differences in recovering sensation as the result of dorsal cell ganglion atrophy, as reported by Koester. The ganglion atrophy and subsequent regrowth, he felt, caused the differences in sensation, rather than Head's observation of two distinct types of sensation.

Head's theory was not initially well supported, though he had carefully documented his work.[7] However, his theory gained popularity after the publication of single unit recordings.[58] Powell and Mountcastle identified specific pathways, lemniscal and spinothalamic, that corresponded to Head's epicritic and protopathic sensation, respectively. These unique pathways are still accepted.[3,60] Nafe's theory refuted receptor specificity, and yet, according to Melzack and Wall, did not propose how the receptors actually functioned within the pattern theory.[53] Nafe, however, continued to emphasize cortical specificity as the key to sensory specificity, and regarded the nerve fibers and sensory receptors only as transmitters of impulse patterns.[58,61-62] Stevens and Green summarized the wide differences of the theories by observing that Nafe's theory is holistic while Von Frey's is specific.[6]

SENSORY TESTING VARIABLES

Many variables come into play during sensory testing, and they can affect the final results of testing. Some can be controlled; others, such as the patient's interpretation of the test, cannot.

The environmental variables, such as interruption, are important to control.[5,52] Some tests, like the Semmes-Weinstein test, require great concentration on the part of the patient, and conversations from other treatments around him make it difficult for the patient to respond. So, choose a small quiet room in which to test.

Temperature can affect the patient's sensibility. Several authors have determined that nerve conduction velocity slows when the temperature drops.[63-66] Therefore, it is important to note the room and skin temperature prior to testing. The room and skin

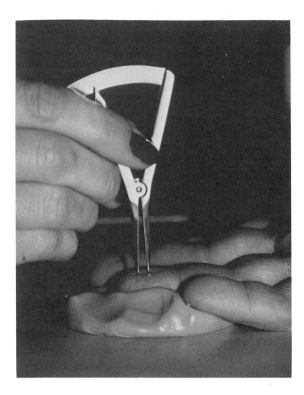

Fig. 3-1. Immobilization of the digit or digits restricts extraneous movements, which can alter sensory test data.

temperature should not drop below 21°C.[63] Allow patients to warm their hands on cool days, before testing, and keep air conditioned rooms from chilling the patient.

During examination, the patient's view needs to be blocked and the tested hand stabilized. Use a table screen or have the patient block his vision during tests. Using a screen prevents the patient from seeing testing instruments and testing records, which can bias results. Cradle the patient's hand or digit in toweling, or preferably putty (Fig. 3-1). If the patient holds the hand in the air, or if the examiner cradles the patient's hand, proprioceptive feedback can be given, which might distort results.

Site selection for testing is a relatively easy variable to control. Some authors choose to test the entire volar surface of the hand.[5,11] However, in this author's experience, enough information can be obtained from careful testing of the volar digital pulp.[52] The digital pulps are the most concentrated areas of receptor density and the portion of the hand most often used for sensory input. Certainly, testing of the entire volar hand is important for monitoring progressive nerve compression or testing of the dorsal hand for radial nerve and ulnar nerve recovery.

Next, the instrument testing tip must be considered. A sharp tip will stimulate pain receptors as well as mechanoreceptors. Instruments, especially those measuring 2PD, have been found to vary in tip width, and will certainly excite different groups of mechanoreceptors, thus provoking different responses. As shown in these detailed figures, the tips of several calipers vary tremendously (Fig. 3-2).

Finally, the administration of the tests is important. The patient should not be prompted by such questions as, "Did you feel that?" or "Can you feel this?" A second

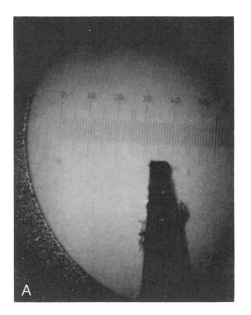

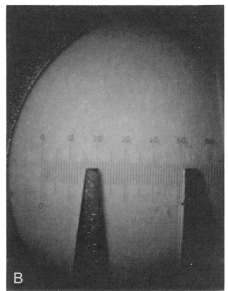

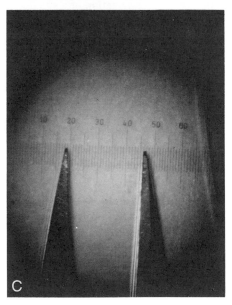

Fig. 3-2. (A) An example of a commercially available two-point discriminator. Tip diameter is .7 mm. Note the ragged rubber edges. (B) An eye caliper that is blunted for use as a two-point discrimination tool. Tip diameter is .4 mm. (C) An eye calipher before blunting. Tip diameter is .1 mm.

form of biasing can occur according to the number of trials performed for each test at each site. If the patient is consistently given two points, then one point during the 2PD test, he can easily guess and be correct in his response 50 percent of the time. A variety of testing methods are available to reduce the likelihood of a biased response. They include forced choice technique, signal detection theory, stimulus masking, methods of profits, and staircase method.[10,39,40,42,49,68–70] What seems most important in reducing test bias is to randomize the test stimulus administration for achieving an accurate set of responses. The third administration variable is the actual administration of the instrument. Force of instrument application with resulting skin pressure has been demonstrated to be inconsistent.[41-43,71] All instruments, except where specified, should be applied perpendicular to the skin surface.

SELECTION OF SENSORY TESTS

One singular test, electrical or manual, does not provide all the information clinicians need when treating peripheral nerve injuries. One test can determine whether abnormal sensation is present, but cannot give information on the quality of the sensation nor the patient's functional sensibility. Popularity of a test does not necessarily mean it is the best test.[71]

Categories of sensory tests are identified, which group similar tests in an orderly fashion. In this manner, the examiner can choose one or two tests from each category and thus have a fairly complete picture of sensory function after testing sessions.

As shown in Table 3-2, the tests are divided into seven categories. Instruments for each test in a category vary; therefore the examiner must keep in mind the potential variables each instrument may present and how those variables will affect results. For a detailed explanation of test administration, the reader is urged to consult the original article describing the test or a general text on this topic. A detailed reference list is provided at the end of the chapter.[4,5,8,10-12,14,16,20,23-25,28,29,32-40,71,72]

Before testing, in the case of nerve lacerations, the regeneration of the nerve should be monitored. Tests are meaningless if no nerve is present. Two ways to monitor regeneration are by plotting the Tinel's sign and by using the ninhydrine test (Fig. 3-3).

Touch

Testing involving touch provides quick information about the presence, absence, or change in the patient's sensibility. Touch tests also identify areas needing sensory testing.[5]

Table 3-2. Sensory Test Categories

Static and Dynamic Spatial Discrimination	Vibration
Two-point discrimination, moving/static[5,12]	Tuning forks[5,32]
(caliper, Boley gauge)	Vibrometer[51]
Renfrew ridge[14]	Optacon[40]
Seniometer[10]	Touch
V-test[67]	Light touch[5]
	Directional touch
Functional or Tactile Gnosis	Pressure
Braile designs[72]	Semmes-Weinstein monofilaments[17,20]
Coin test[18]	Localization
Moberg pick-up test[16]	Monofilament localization[5,23,24]
Block test[28]	Sudomotor
Size discrimination test[35]	Ninhydrine test[14,35]
Edshage arrow test[29]	Wrinkle test[33,34]

Superscript numbers refer to references.

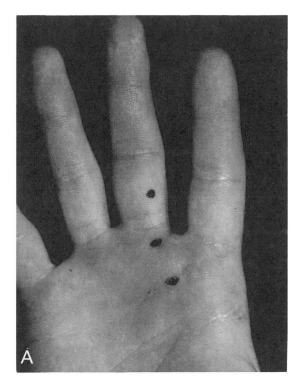

Fig. 3-3. (A) The plotting of the Tinel's sign of the radial digital nerve. The most proximal dot indicates the repair site; the two distal dots indicate regeneration of the nerve. (B) A ninhydrin test used to obtain additional information of radial and ulnar digital nerve loss of the index digit secondary to infection.

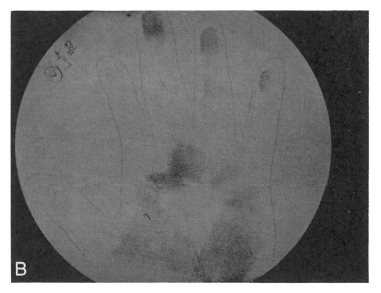

Vibration

As pointed out by Bell, the use of tuning forks provides an inconsistent stimulus to the patient.[73] The amplitude of the vibration frequency is not held constant as the tuning fork is applied. Even in the alternative method by Dellon, the tuning fork is still not providing consistent stimuli.[32] The Bio-thesiometer, however, provides constant vibration at 120 c/s with the change of the stimulus delivered measured in microns of relative amplitude.[51] Thus, small changes in vibration threshold can be measured, which is important in identifying stages of nerve compression.[48,50,51]

Static and Dynamic Spatial Discrimination

These tests provide information about the number of slowly adapting and rapidly adapting mechanoreceptors found within an area tested.[74,75] Weber in 1845 and later Gibson in 1962 cited how a tested individual[8,76] can perceive a stimulus more often if actively touched rather than statically touched. Many different instruments (paper clip, Boley gauge, caliper) have been suggested for testing static and moving 2PD. Again the examiner must weight the instrument variables and how they will affect the test results. This author prefers an eye caliper blunted to .4 mm for this testing, which will consistently stimulate the patient's skin. No barbs or variations in tip width can affect the test results. The two ridge devices (Sensiometer, Renfrew ridge) can be used for quick assessment of the same parameters.

Pressure

Light touch/deep pressure, as these tests are often called, provide important information about the threshold of the mechanoreceptors within the testing area. Studies have shown that this information demonstrates relative nerve compression as well as recovery status after nerve regeneration.

Localization

Localization, by utilizing the Semmes-Weinstein monofilaments and a small dowel, is useful in noting the extent of nerve recovery and the effectiveness of sensory re-education.

Functional Tests or Tactile Gnosis

Function is the key word in sensibility. While the patient may have acceptable test measurements of, say, 2PD, if he cannot use his hand for everyday activities, he does not have a functional result, only an academic result. Many tests are available, as noted in Table 3-2, to assess how the patient uses the sensation he has.

Sudomotor

Sympathetic nervous system function can indicate sensory change or loss. However, sudomotor test cannot be used only to assess sensory status, as we discussed in the beginning of this section. These tests are helpful to monitor nerve regeneration, to evaluate malingers and to test small children, as they do not require patient participation.

INTERPRETATION OF SENSORY TESTING

In the sections of this chapter's introduction and historical perspective, one gathers that there are many ways to interpret sensory test batteries. Again, the reader is urged to gather data from several tests in the different categories to provide a more complete picture. Second, the patient's contralateral hand is tested to serve as the guide for that patient's normal sensibility. Keep in mind that the information may be abnormal in patients with systemic disease or suspected bilateral nerve compression. Third, use the many tables available for assessment of test results.[5,8,11,23,24,26] Fourth, compare your sensory test findings with sensory nerve conduction results. If the patient is suspected of having median nerve compression, do your findings coincide with the nerve conduction reports. Fifth, keep in mind several other variables that can affect the outcome of your sensory testing, such as primary versus secondary repair, wound status, site of injury, infection, patient's age, and patient's occupation.

SENSORY RE-EDUCATION

Numerous investigators have documented the poor quality of sensibility that returns to the hand following peripheral nerve repair in the adult. Although children recover well,[77-79,80] the typical result in the adult is fair to good return of pain, temperature, and touch perception, but poor return of localization, two-point discrimination, tactile gnosis, and other measures of functional sensation.[71,80-83]

The level of functional sensation is poor, because regeneration is imperfect. Several factors that contribute to imperfect regeneration have been noted by Sunderland.[87] These include: (1) Retrograde damage to the parent neuron that occurs as a result of damage to the nerve trunk. The higher the level of the initial injury, the greater the damage to the parent cell, and the greater the negative effect on diameter and number of regenerating axons. (2) Scar tissue at the suture site inhibits successful crossing of the suture site by regenerating axons. Depending upon the amount and density of the scar, an individual axon will successfully cross the suture site, or it may "dead-end" and double back into the proximal stump, or turn laterally and terminate in connective tissues outside the nerve. (3) Once across the suture site, the axon must successfully re-enter a funiculus (a bundle of axons ensheathed by perineurium), but it may fail to do so and terminate instead in the connective tissue between funiculi. (4) Within a funiculus there is, usually, a combination of motor, sensory, and sympathetic fibers. Each fiber has its own endoneurial sheath. The regenerating sensory axon must enter a sheath that formerly was occupied by a sensory axon. Even if it manages to do so, it will probably not enter the same sheath as it occupied previously, and therefore the spatial or somatotopic organization of the nerve fibers will be altered. (5) Finally, the regenerating axon must successfully reinnervate a sensory end organ which will have undergone some atrophy.

The final result of regeneration is fewer and smaller diameter nerve fibers and an altered somatotopic organization of fibers. Horch[84] has stated that the effect on function of fewer and smaller nerve fibers may not be as significant as was previously thought, because that deficit may be less than that which occurs naturally during the aging process. The effect of the disturbed somatotopic organization is of undisputed significance. It means that when a stimulus occurs at the periphery, the pattern of impulses that travels to the brain will differ from the pre-injury pattern. Functionally, this results in deficits in localization, two-point discrimination, and ability to recognize texture and shape, even in the presence of normal or near normal perception of pain, temperature, and touch. Thus, even though the patient may perceive that his hand is touching something cold and sharp, he will not know what that object is.

Can Functional Sensation Be Improved in the Adult Hand?

At this time it is not clear to what extent functional sensation can be retrained in the adult following nerve repair, but it is clear that some improvement is possible. Clinicians have noted for many years that two people with the same level of nerve injury and return of sensation, as measured clinically, may demonstrate very different levels of function in their nerve injured hands. The higher level of function was attributed by Stopford[79] to a period of "reeducation" in a "capable patient." Davis,[85] Bowden,[86] Onne,[25] and others[84,87] all noted the role of motivation, persistent use of the extremity, and learning in helping one person to overcome a sensory deficit, while another of lesser motivation and trainability does not overcome the deficit. These observations were made even without the benefit of a formal re-education program.

Rationale for Sensory Re-education Program

When sensory reeducation programs have been formally administered, the results have been good.[30,88,89] The rationale for a formal sensory re-education program is that the motivated patient who has a sensory deficit can be trained by making use of learning principles (i.e., attention, feedback, memory, and reinforcement) to maximize function in the hand. The fact that fibers are fewer and smaller and disorganized relative to the pre-injury state cannot be changed. However, the patient can learn to correctly decode the altered messages sent to the brain. Structured, formal training sessions speed up and maximize the "re-education" process noted earlier by Stopford[79] and others.

Typically, in a formal re-education session, the patient is given a sensory task while his vision is occluded. He might be asked to identify the location of a touch or identify a texture. If he is successful, he is informed of such and given a different task. If unsuccessful, he is instructed to open his eyes and observe the repetition of the stimulus, thus integrating vision with tactile experience. Finally, he is instructed to close his eyes again, and the stimulus is repeated for reinforcement, as he integrates his visual memory of the stimulus with his present experience of it. Attention is maximized by training in a quiet room and limiting the session to 10 to 15 minutes, 1 to 3 times a day. Daily practice sessions reinforce the learning. These training techniques have been used with success by Wynn Parry[88,89] and Dellon.[30,91]

Prerequisites for Training

Candidates for training in discriminative sensory re-education must have return of protective sensation and touch perception to the fingertips. The latter can be assessed by the use of a graded light touch–deep pressure test instrument,*[.90] or, more grossly, by the patient's ability to perceive the touch of the examiner's fingertip. Of equal importance, the patient must be motivated, intelligent, able to concentrate, and willing to work daily to achieve his goal.

Methods of Training

Training is divided into two main categories: localization and graded discrimination.[5] Both categories of tasks are included in the program from start to finish.

Training in Localization. The patient's eyes are closed, and he concentrates as the fingertip of the examiner lightly touches, with a moving or stationary touch,[30] a small area of skin. The patient is then asked to open his eyes and point to the spot stimulated. If correct, he closes his eyes and waits for the application of another stimulus. If incorrect, he is instructed to watch as the stimulus is reapplied to the same spot, and then closes his eyes and concentrates as the stimulus is applied once more. This process is continued over the entire area of involvement. These methods are common to other formal programs.[30,88,89,91]

Training in Discrimination. Activities should be graded in difficulty and designed so that they can be carried out independently by the patient, thereby reducing therapist time and patient dependence on another person at home. Early in the program, if motor dysfunction is significant, activities are chosen that do not require advanced motor skills. Each task uses the eyes closed, eyes open, eyes closed sequence, with feedback and repetition for reinforcement.

Texture and Shape Discrimination Tasks.

1. Texture discrimination using sandpaper or other textures on dowels. A coarse grade of sandpaper is attached to one end of several dowels. On the opposite end is attached either the same coarse grade or a different grade, varying from coarse to extra fine. First one end of a selected dowel, then the other end, is lightly moved over a small area of skin while the patient's eyes are closed. He is asked whether the two ends are the same or different. If incorrect, he watches while the stimuli are applied again to the same area, and then closes his eyes while they are applied once again. If correct, training proceeds to a different area. As discrimination improves, the grades of sandpaper chosen for practice become more similar.

The textures are attached to dowels so the patient can carry out the activity independently and without inadvertently providing sensory cues to uninvolved surfaces (Fig. 3-4). After evaluation, the therapist selects certain dowels for training. Working alone and with his eyes closed, the patient picks up a dowel at the center and applies first one end then the other to an involved area. After answering the question, "Are these the same or different?," he opens his eyes to check himself. If incorrect, he

---

* Semmes-Weinstein Pressure Aesthesiometer. Research Designs Inc, 7320 Ashcroft, Suite 103, Houston, TX 77081.

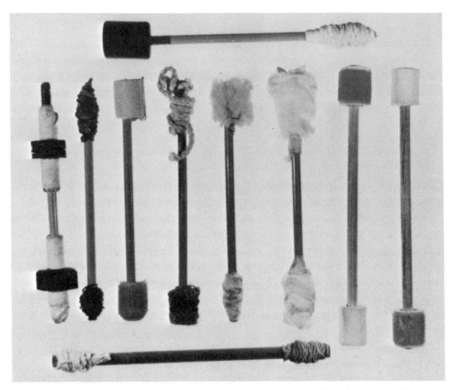

Fig. 3-4.   Textures are attached to dowels so the patient can perform the task independently, without providing cues to uninvolved sensory surfaces. (Callahan AD: Methods of compensation and reeducation for sensory dysfunction. In Hunter JM et al (eds): Rehabilitation of the hand. 2nd Ed. CV Mosby Co, St Louis, 1984)

reapplies both ends while watching and concentrates on what he is feeling, then repeats the step with eyes closed. He then puts down the dowel, with eyes closed, "shuffles" the dowels, and repeats the process with a newly selected dowel.

2. Texture discrimination using fabrics. At first the patient is required simply to "match" a texture with one from a small group of possibilities. Later, the group of possibilities is enlarged, and he is required to identify the fabric.

This activity can be carried out independently if the textures are attached to cards in a "book" with a circular binding. Then, with his eyes closed, the patient matches fabrics selected for training with those in the book (Fig. 3-5).

3. Differentiation of rough and smooth edges of coins, nuts, and bolts. Dellon[30,91] has recommended that the patient carry these objects in a pocket for frequent training sessions.

Games and Puzzles.   Games and puzzles are used to provide more interest and challenge to the patient. Described below are some examples.

1. Letter identification. Block letters formed from adhesive hook Velcro* are

---

* Velcro. Velcro USA, Inc, 681 Fifth Ave, New York, NY 10022

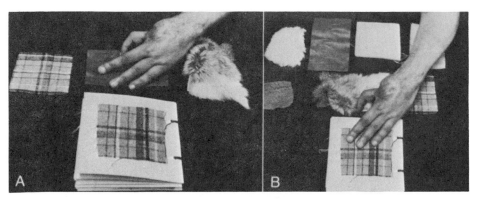

Fig. 3-5. (A,B) Patient is required to match the test fabrics with those in the "book". The activity is designed so that it can be carried out independently by the patient. (Callahan AD: Methods of compensation and reeducation for sensory dysfunction. In Hunter JM et al (eds.): Rehabilitation of the Hand. 2nd Ed. CV Mosby Co, St Louis, 1984)

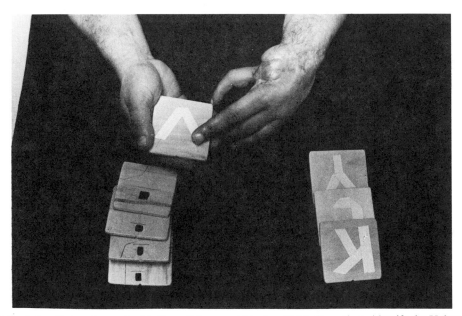

Fig. 3-6. Patient is required to "scan" the wood block with his fingertip to identify the Velcro letter. (Callahan AD: Methods of compensation and reeducation for sensory dysfunction. In Hunter JM et al (eds.): Rehabilitation of the Hand. 2nd Ed. CV Mosby Co, St Louis, 1984)

made to adhere to small square wood blocks. The patient must identify the letter by "scanning" over the Velcro with his fingertip (Fig. 3-6). A time limit can be used to make this more challenging to the patient.

If there is sufficient motor return to enable manipulation, then three-dimensional letters cut out of wood are recommended to make the task more difficult.

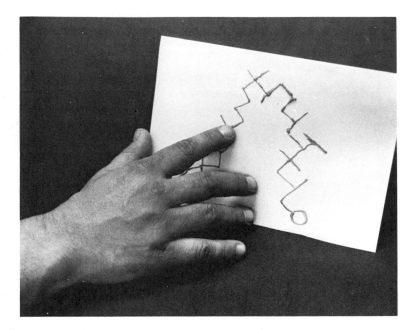

Fig. 3-7. Finger mazes provide a challenge to the patient. (Callahan AD: Methods of compensation and reeducation for sensory dysfunction. In Hunter JM et al (eds.): Rehabilitation of the Hand. 2nd Ed. CV Mosby Co, St Louis, 1984.)

2. Braille designs. Millesi[72] and Walsh[92] have described the use of braille designs in retraining. Using Walsh's approach, a braille design, such as a house, is imprinted on braille paper and presented to the patient whose eyes are closed. He is then given a task, such as "Determine the number of windows." Depending upon how closely spaced the components of the design are, this task can be made easier or more difficult.

3. Finger mazes. "Puzzles" are devised by using a colored epoxy* to form a raised maze on cardboard. Vision is occluded, and the patient is instructed to place his fingertip at the start of the maze (designated by some geometric shape) and trace his way to a finishing point (designated by some other geometric shape) (Fig. 3-7).

Tasks That Require Motor Function. The following tasks require more advanced motor skills. These, too, can be graded in difficulty, and if motor function is adequate, they can be prescribed concurrently with the above tasks.

1. Picking up objects from a background medium of rice, sand, styrofoam, chips, etc. At first, large objects are used, progressing to tiny objects that are similar in size to the background medium.

2. Identification of common objects. Everyday items are placed into a "grab bag." Initially, objects are chosen because they are dissimilar, but later, they are chosen because of similarity in size, shape, or texture.

3. Activities of daily living and work-stimulated activities. Many self-care and work activities require manipulation of an object without the aid of direct vision. Therefore, these activities form an important part of training (Fig. 3-8).

---

* Hi-Marks. Mark-Tex Corp, Englewood, NJ.

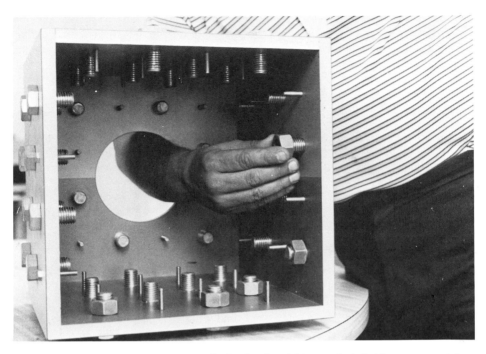

Fig. 3-8.   As motor skills improve, work-simulated activities are included in sensory training. (Callahan AD: Methods of compensation and reeducation for sensory dysfunction. In Hunter JM et al (eds.): Rehabilitation of the Hand. 2nd Ed. CV Mosby Co, St Louis, 1984.)

Selection of Activities

The exact choice of activity depends upon evaluation of baseline discrimination skill, including two-point discrimination, localization, an ADL interview to determine specific problem areas, and brief trials in some of the above activities. Training sessions should be brief, approximately 10 to 15 minutes, because good concentration is required. At least one session should be carried out daily, but two or three sessions are ideal. Each session should include practice and training in localization, texture discrimination, a puzzle or game, and a task that requires integration of motor and sensory function. The therapist designs the program and provides feedback to the patient; the patient gives feedback to the therapist about relative difficulty of tasks and the cues he uses to help perform tasks.

Assessment of Results

Assessment of results of sensory re-education cannot be done precisely. Some clinically useful parameters include: (1) Notation of fewer errors in localization. (2) Increased number of accurate responses. More objects or textures are matched or identified in a given time period. Note: different items should be used for evaluation than are used for training. (3) Time required to complete a task becomes shorter. (4) Improvement in two-point discrimination. Though this is a commonly used measure of improvement in sensory function,[30,81] some argue that it is not a valid measure of function after nerve repair.[29,88] (5) Patient report of increased function in ADL and work activities. The most important measure of success is the patient's increased ability to use his hand in work and leisure activities.

Long Term Effects

Maintenance of gains made in sensory re-education depends upon continued use of the hand after formal training stops.[25,85,78] The level of discrimination required in the patient's daily activities will determine whether function improves even further or diminishes with time.[89]

SUMMARY

The rationale for a formal sensory re-education program is that a person can learn through attention, feedback, integration, and recall to enhance sensory function after nerve repair. Such re-education requires that the patient have a certain level of sensory return and that he be intelligent, motivated, and willing to make a conscious effort to incorporate the hand into activities of daily living and to carry out structured sensory tasks. Maintenance of gains will depend on persistent use of the hand after training steps. The effectiveness of sensory re-education has been demonstrated, but further studies are needed to determine the most efficient approach and to better define its capabilities.

REFERENCES

1. Wolf S, Nahai F, Brown D, Jordan N, Kutner M: Objective determination of sensibility in the upper extremity: Part I—Median nerve sensory conduction velocities. Phys Ther 57: 1121, 1977
2. Omer G: Sensibility of the hand as opposed to sensation in the hand. Ann Chir 27:479, 1973
3. Mountcastle V: Sensory receptors and neural coding: Introduction to sensory processes. In Mountcastle V (ed): Medical Physiology. 14th Ed. CV Mosby, St Louis, 1980
4. Weinstein S: Intensive and extensive aspects of tactile sensitivity as a function of body part, sex and laterality. In Kenshalo D (ed): The Skin Senses: *Proceedings of the First International Symposium on Skin Senses*. C Thomas Co Springfield, 1968
5. Callahan A: Sensibility testing: Clinical methods. In Hunter JM et al (eds): Rehabilitation of the Hand. 2nd ed. CV Mosby Co, St Louis, 1984
6. Stevens J, Green B: History of Research in Feeling. In Caterette, E, Friedman M (eds): Handbook of Perception. Vol. 6B. Academic Press, New York, 1978
7. Sinclair C: The Major Theories. In Cutaneous Sensation, University Press London, 1967
8. Weber E: The sense of Touch, Ross H, Murray D (trans). Academic Press London, 1978
9. Johansson R, Vallbo A: Detection of tactile stimuli: Thresholds of afferent units related to psychophysical thresholds in the human hand. J Physiol 297:405, 1979
10. Poppen N, McCarroll R, Doyle J, Niebayer J: Sensibility after suture of digitial nerves. J Hand Surg 4:212, 1979

11. Bell J: Sensibility Evaluation. In Hunter J, Schneider L, Mackin E, Bell J (eds): Rehabilitation of the Hand. CV Mosby Co, St Louis, 1978
12. Dellon AL: The moving 2PD test. J Hand Surg 3:474, 1978
13. Dellon AL: Reinnervation of dennervated Meissner corpuscles: a sequential histologic study in the monkey following fascicular repair. J Hand Surg 1:98, 1976
14. Renfrew S: Finger-tip sensation, A routine neurological test. Lancet Feb 22:396, 1969
15. Moberg E: Methods of Examining Sensibility of the Hand. In Flynn J (ed): Hand Surgery 2nd Ed. Williams & Wilkins, Baltimore, 1975
16. Moberg E: Objective method for determining the functional value of sensibility in the hand. J Bone Joint Surg 40B: 454, 1958
17. Von Frey M: The distribution of afferent nerves in the skin. JAMA 47: 645, 1906
18. Seddon H: War injuries of peripheral nerves. Br J Surg 2:325, 1949
19. Bunnell S: Surgery of the Hand. 5th Ed. Boyes J (ed): JB Lippincott Co, Philadelphia, 1944
20. Weinstein S: Tactile sensitivity of the phalanges. Percept Mot Skills 14:351, 1962
21. Weinstein S, Sersen E: Tactual sensitivity as a function of handedness and laterality. J Comp Physiol Psychol 54:665, 1961
22. Von Prince K: Measurement of sensory function following injury. Read to Symposium on Assessment of Levels of Cutaneous Sensation, Carville, LA, 1980
23. Von Prince K, Butler B: Measuring sensory function of the hand in peripheral nerve injuries. Am J Occup Ther 21:385, 1967
24. Werner J, Omer G: Evaluating cutaneous pressure sensation of the hand. Am J Occup Ther 24:347, 1970
25. Onne L: Recovery of sensibility and sudomotor activity in the hand after nerve sutures. Acta Chir Scand, Suppl 300:1, 1962
26. Flynn J, Flynn W: Median and ulnar injury: Long range study with evaluation of ninhydrine test, sensory and motor returns. Ann Surg 156:1002, 1962
27. Renfrew S, Melville I: The somantic sense of space and its threshold, brain. J Neurol 83:93, 1960
28. Porter R: New test for fingertip sensation. Br Med J 2:927, 1966
29. Edshage S: Experience with Clinical Methods of Testing Sensation after Peripheral Nerve Surgery. In Jewett D, McCarroll H (eds): Nerve Repair and Regeneration. CV Mosby Co, St Louis, 1980
30. Dellon AL, Curtis R, Edgerton M: Evaluating recovery of sensation in the hand following nerve injury. Hopkins Med J 130:235, 1972
31. Dellon AL: The paper clip: Light hardware to evaluate sensibility in the hand. Contemp Orthop 1:23, 1979
32. Dellon AL: Clinical use of vibratory stimuli to evaluate peripheral nerve injury and compression neuropathy. Plast Reconstr Surg 65:466, 1980
33. Phelps P, Walker E: Comparison of the finger wrinkling test results to established sensory tests in peripheral nerve injury. Am J Occup Ther 3:565, 1977
34. O'Riain S: New and simple test of nerve function in the hand. Br Med J 3:615, 1973
35. Guttman L: Topographic studies of disturbances of sweat secretion after complete lesions of peripheral nerves. J Neuro Psychiatry 3:197, 1940
36. Vierck C, Jones M: Size discrimination on the skin. Science 163:488, 1969
37. Kanatani F: A comparative engineering study of the Semmes-Weinstein nylon filament pressure anesthesiometer and the prototype steel wire pressure anesthesiometer. Unpublished material, 1979
38. Carlson W, Shlomo S, Taylor W, Wessterman D: Instrumentation for measurement of sensory loss in the fingertips. J Occup Med 21:260, 1974
39. Craig J: Vibrotactile letter recognition: The effects of a masking stimulus. Perception 20: 317, 1976

40. Arezzo J, Schaumburg H: The use of the optacon as a screening device. J Occup Med 22:461, 1980
41. Dyck P, O'Brien P, Bushek W, Oviatt K, Schilling K, Steven J: Clinical vs. quantitative evaluation of cutaneous sensation. Arch Neurol 33:651 1976
42. Dyck P: Properties of assessment methods. Read to Symposium on Assessment of Levels of Cutaneous Sensation, Carville LA, 1980
43. Dyck P, Zimmerman I, O'Brien P, et al: Introduction of automated systems to evaluate touch-pressure, vibration and thermal cutaneous sensation in man. Ann Neurol 4:502, 1978
44. DeMichels F, Giaretti W, Barberis M, Simon T: Biomedical instrumentation for the measurements of skin sensitivity. IEEE Trans Biomed Eng 26:326, 1979
45. Looft F, Williams W: On-line receptive field mapping of cutaneous receptors. IEEE Trans Biomed Eng 26:350, 1979
46. Levin S, Pearsall G, Ruderman R: Von Frey's method of measuring pressure sensibility in the hand: An engineering analysis of Semmes-Weinstein pressure anesthesiometer. J Hand Surg 3:211, 1978
47. Chockinov R, Ullyot L, Moorhouse J: Sensory perception thresholds in patients with juvenile diabetes and their close relatives. N Engl J Med 286:1233, 1972
48. Gregarson G: Vibratory perception threshold and motor conduction velocity in diabetic and non-diabetics. Acta Med Scand 183:61, 1968
49. Heinrich R, Moorhouse J: Touch perception thresholds in blind diabetic subjects in relation to the reading of braille type. N Engl J Med 280:72, 1969
50. Lundborg G et al: Median nerve compression in the carpal tunnel—Functional response to explain induced controlled pressure. J Hand Surg 7:252, 1982
51. Szabo RM et al: Vibratory sensory testing in acute peripheral nerve compression. J Hand Surg 9A: 104, 1984
52. Moran CA: Comparison of sensory testing methods using carpal tunnel syndrome patients. Unpublished Master's Thesis, Medical College of Virginia/Virginia Commonwealth University, 1981
53. Melzack R, Wall P: On the nature of cutaneous sensory mechanisms. Brain, J Neurol 85: 331, 1962
54. Brown E, Deffenbacher K: Perception and the senses. Oxford Univer Pr Inc, New York, 1979
55. Boring E: Sensation and Perception in The History of Experimental Psychology. Elliott R (ed): Appleton-Crofts, Inc, New York, 1942
56. Head H: Studies in Neurology. Oxford Univ Pr Inc, London, 1920
57. Sherrington D: Cutaneous Sensations. In Schafer E (ed): Textbook of Physiology. Vol. 2, Young Pentland Company, Edinburgh, 1900
58. Nafe J, Wagnor K: The Nature of Pressure Adaptation. J Gen Psychol 25:323, 1941
59. Powell T, Mountcastle V: Some aspect of the functional organization of the cortex of the post-central gyrus of the monkey: A correlation of findings obtained in single unit analysis with cytoarchitecture. Bull John's Hopkins Hosp 105:133, 1949
60. Zimmerman M: Neurophysiology of the Sensory System. In Schmidt R (ed): Fundamentals of Sensory Physiology. Springer-Verlag New York Inc 1978
61. Nafe J: Neural Correlates of Sensation. In Kenshalo D (ed): The Skin Senses. Proceedings of the First International Symposium on Skin Senses. CC Thomas Co, Springfield, 1968
62. Nafe J: A Quantitative Theory of Feeling, J Gen Psychol 1-2:199, 1928
63. de Jesus P, Hausmanow-Petruse-Wics I, Barchi R: The effect of cold on nerve conduction of human slow and fast nerve fibers. Neurology 23:1182, 1973

64. Abramson D, Hlavova A, Rickert B et al: Effect of ischemia on latencies of the median nerve in the hand at various temperatures. Arch Phys Med Rehabil 51:471, 1970
65. Abramson D et al: Effect of ischemia on median and ulnar nerve conduction velocities at various temperatures. Arch Phys Med Rehabil 51:463, 1970
66. Buchthal F, Rosenfolck A: Evoked action potentials and conduction velocity in human sensory nerves. Brain Res 3:1, 1966
67. Mackworth N: Finger numbness in very cold winds. J Appl Physiol 5:533, 1952
68. Knibestol M, Vallbo A: Intensity of sensation related to activity of SA mechanoreceptor units in the human hand. J Physiol 300:251, 1980
69. Wolf S, Cohen B: Sensory threshold measurements for electrical stimulation of the digits. Arch Phys Med Rehabil 58:127, 1977
70. Clark W: Pain sensitivity and the report of pain. Anesthiology 40:272, 1974
71. Bell J: Sensibility Testing: State of the Art. In Hunter J H et al (eds): Rehabilitation of the Hand. CV Mosby Co, St. Louis, 1984
72. Millesi H, Rinderer C: A method for training and testing sensibility in the fingertips. The Department of Plastic and Reconstructive Surgery, Surgical University Clinic of Vienna and Ludwig-Boltzmann Inst for Experimental Plastic Surgery, Australia, 1978
73. Bell J, Buford W: The force/time relationship of clinically used sensory testing instruments. Presented to the American Society for Surgery of the Hand in New Orleans, LA, 1982
74. Johansson R, Vallbo A: The density of mechanoreceptors and the spatial discriminative capacity in the human hand. Acta Physiol Scand, Suppl 400:81, 1976
75. Johansson R: Receptive field sensitivity profile of mechanosensitive units innervating the glabrous skin of the human hand. Brain Res 104:330, 1976
76. Gibson J: Observations on active touch. Psychol Rev 69:477, 1962
77. Almquist E, Eeg-Olofsson O: Sensory nerve conduction velocity and two-point discrimination in sutured nerves. J Bone Joint Surg 52-A: 791, 1970
78. Omer GE: Sensory evaluation by the pick-up test. In Jewett, DL, McCarroll HK, Jr, and Relton H, (eds): Nerve Repair and Regeneration: Its Clinical and Experimental Basis. CV Mosby Co, St Louis, 1979
79. Stopford JSB: An explanation of the two-stage recovery of sensation during regeneration of a peripheral nerve. Brain 49:372, 1926
80. Forster FM, Shields CD: Cortical sensory deficitis causing disability. Arch Phys Med Rehabil 40:56, 1959
81. Reid RL: Preliminary results of sensibility re-education following repair of median nerve. American Society for Surgery of the Hand, Newsletter #15, 1977
82. Stromberg WB, McFarlane RM, Bell JL et al: Injury of the median and ulnar nerves: One hundred and fifty cases with an evaluation of Moberg's ninhydrin test. J Bone Joint Surg 43-A:717, 1961
83. Sperry RW: The problem of central nervous reorganization after nerve regeneration and muscle transposition. Q Rev Biol 20:311, 1945
84. Horch KW, Burgess PR: Functional specificity and somatotopic organization during peripheral nerve regeneration. In Jewett DL, McCarroll HK, Jr, Relton H (eds): Nerve Repair and Regeneration: Its Clinical and Experimental Basis. CV Mosby Co, St Louis, 1979
85. Davis DR: Some factors affecting the results of treatment of peripheral nerve injuries. Lancet 1:877, 1949
86. Bowden REM: Factors influencing functional recovery. In Seddon HJ (ed): Peripheral Nerve Injuries. Her Majesty's Stationery Office, London, 1954
87. Sunderland S: Nerves and nerve injuries. 2nd Ed. Churchill Livingstone, New York, 1978

88. Wynn Parry CB: Rehabilitation of the Hand. 2nd Ed. Butterworths, London, 1973
89. Wynn Parry CB, Salter M: Sensory re-education after median nerve lesion. Hand 8:250, 1976
90. Bell JA: Light touch/deep pressure testing using the Semmes-Weinstein monofilaments. In Hunter JH et al (eds): Rehabilitation of the Hand. 2nd Ed. CV Mosby Co, St Louis, 1984
91. Dellon AL: Evaluation of Sensibility and Re-education of Sensation in the Hand. Williams & Wilkins, Baltimore, 1981
92. Walsh WW: Sensory modalities v functional use approach to re-education. Presented at: Symposium: Assessment of Levels of Cutaneous Sensibility. USPHS Hospital, Carville, LA, September, 1980
93. Hawkins GE: Faulty sensory localization in nerve regeneration. J Neurosurg 5:11, 1948
94. Omer GE: Sensation and sensibility in the upper extremity. Clin Orthop 104:30, 1974
95. Vinograd A, Taylor E, Grossman S: Sensory retraining of the hemiplegic hand. Am J Occup Ther 5:246, 1962

4 | Conservative Management of Vasospastic Diseases

Heather L. Delp

Vasomotor disabilities occur as a result of direct trauma, systemic disease, and occupational hazards, and can affect people from all walks of life. Most often these disorders are classified as reflex sympathetic dystrophy (RSD), Raynaud's disease or phenomenon (RD or RP).

Men at war injured by a sniper's gun, women with scleroderma, jackhammer or chainsaw operators, and truck drivers who have the dorsum of their hand struck by an object are all possible victims of RSDS or RP. In the past a large part of their treatment consisted of surgical procedures or drug therapy, but recently, physical therapists have taken a more active role in the rehabilitation of these patients. The purpose of this chapter is to:

1. Expound on the etiological theories of these syndromes,
2. Review pertinent anatomical features,
3. Present a method of clinical examination and assessment skills,
4. Offer a treatment repertoire.

A description of reflex sympathetic dystrophy syndrome (RSD) and Raynaud's phenomenon (RP) was first reported in the literature of the mid 1800s.[1,2] Since then, the use of these and other similar terms has been confused. To describe vasospastic disorders, RSD has been proposed as a "catch-all" phrase for those disabilities whose signs and symptoms suggest vasomotor instability with associated pain, swelling, and tenderness.[3] Other commonly used expressions have included causalgia, post-traumatic sympathetic dystrophy, Sudeck's atrophy, sympathalgia, shoulder-hand syndrome, and post-traumatic painful osteoporosis.

The same nomenclature problems exist when identifying Raynaud's phenomenon. Terms such as Raynaud's disease, primary Raynaud's, and secondary Raynaud's have been indiscriminately used to describe the symptoms of triphasic digital skin discolorations. This phenomenon, RP, does not suggest etiology. Primary Raynaud's should be used to identify individuals who exhibit the phenomenon symmetrically and bilaterally, without associated disease or injury.[4] Secondary Raynaud's is defined as RP occurring concurrently with one of the following entities: (1) cold injury, (2) the use of a vibratory tool, (3) an endocrine disorder, (4) arterial disease, (5) arterial compression, (6) collagen disease, or (7) blood disorders.[5,6] All of the above are precipitated by cold exposure, but primary RP can also be the result of emotional stress.[7,8]

ETIOLOGY

A common thread between RSD and primary and secondary RP or RD is that in both diagnoses altered blood flow to the extremity occurs, with resultant pain; the pain of RP follows cold exposure. The normal response to local cooling of short duration is vasoconstriction, and the proposed mechanisms responsible for the vascular response have been reported by Folkow et al.[9] To create the initial reaction of vasoconstriction, the four factors are considered to be: (1) reflex sympathetic fiber excitation, (2) smooth muscle contraction, (3) an increase in blood viscosity, and (4) a local chemical change with a resultant increase in vasomotor tone.

Altered hemodynamics contribute to exaggerated vasoconstriction in persons with secondary RP. A reduction in blood volume due to a decrease in lumen diameter, an increase in blood viscosity, or a change in the pressure gradient along a vessel wall can all be responsible for the changes in digital skin color people with secondary RP experience. Arterial obstruction and stenosis due to connective tissue disease have been visualized by the use of arteriograms[10,11] and by muscle biopsy.[12] Porter et al not only described occluded vessels in these patients, but also noted digital vasospasms.[10] Another cause of decreased blood flow can be vasculitis, as is found in rheumatoid arthritis. According to Scott and colleagues, RA leads to collagenous intimal thickening.[13] Hypertrophy of smooth muscle due to the use of pneumatic hammers has been cited as a cause of secondary Raynaud's. It has been theorized that distention of vessels caused by vibration eventually leads to smooth muscle hypertrophy and a reduced lumen size.[14] When presented with a cold stimulus, vasoconstriction is exaggerated, because the vessel is already partially occluded. Cross sections of hypertrophied arterial walls have been discovered in some vibratory tool users.[15] An increase in blood viscosity upon cooling is the cause of Raynaud's in persons with cold agglutinins syndrome,[16] cryoglobulinemias, and cryofibrinogenemias.[17]

When treating patients with RP, the cause of their decreased blood flow should be considered. Not all of the above-mentioned conditions benefit from all types of treatments for Raynaud's phenomenon. For example, Johnston et al[18] noted poor results in sympathectomy for patients with advanced scleroderma. Obliteration of sympathetic tone will allow vasodilatation, but only to the limit of the occluded vessel. Perhaps the treatment of these patients should be aimed at lysing fibrin deposits and reducing their blood viscosity. Fibrolytic enhancers have been reported to successfully reduce ischemic pain by improving the volume of blood flow.[19,20]

Reduction in blood flow is also a cause of primary RP, but its pathogenesis is nebulous. One theory states that the sympathetic nervous system is hyperirritable, leading to an exaggerated response to a cold stimulus. Abolishing sympathectic control through peripheral nerve anesthesization[21] and sympathectomies[22] decreases the occurrence of cold-induced RP. Also, activation of the sympathetic system by emotional stress has been cited as a cause of RP.[8] Typical symptoms of pain, pallor, and cyanosis have been demonstrated during stressful situations.

The second theory of blood flow reduction claims that obstruction of the vessels does not exist and that the sympathetic system is not responsible for vasospasms. Rather, the digital vessels alone are the cause of the abnormal response to cold. A reduction in the plethysmographic blood flow at warm and cold temperatures,[23,24] a significant difference in finger systolic pressure between controlled and primary Raynaud's patients,[25] and evidence that the central thermoregulatory system is functioning normally[26] substantiates that theory. The type of treatment recommended is based on the acceptance of one theory or the other. For example, sympathetic blocks, axillary or digital artery sympathetomies would not be the preferential treatment chosen by those who believe that pathology is inherent to the digital vessels.

RSD Theories

As with primary RP, several theories exist to explain the vasomotor instability of RSD. Pain, swelling, trophic changes of an upper or lower extremity can be preceded by numerous types of injury. Associated conditions include: fractures, herniated discs, myocardial infarction, cerebral vascular accident, herpes zoster, thrombophlebitis, trauma, and idiopathy.[27] As the theories of RSD are described, the types of related diagnoses should be remembered, as some theories are supported by certain diagnoses and others are not.

Livingston's theory (as reported by Steinbrocker[28] and Drucker et al.), the "internuncial pool" theory, requires that three neurological criteria be met. First, prolonged irritation of a peripheral nerve due to tissue damage or trauma must be present. This chronic state increases the number of afferent impulses being generated to the spinal cord. Secondly, these sensory messages that travel to the dorsal columns must be spread between interconnecting neurons of the same and adjacent segments. Then, the stimuli is again transmitted by internuncial neurons to the vasomotor and anterior horn cells. Thirdly, prolonged and heightened stimulation of these motor and sympathetic neurons occurs, leading to symptoms of pain, edema, and muscle spasm. These conditions then further irritate the tissues, and a vicious cycle is born, which perpetuates itself. When commenting on a similar theory, Sunderland[29] refutes this proposal because it does not explain the immediate pain perceived by some causalgia patients. Pathology, he states, requires time to develop.

Whereas, Livingston's theory specified an abnormal sympathetic reflex, Doupe[1] and Zimmerman[30] described an "artificial synapse" or ephase, between efferent sympathetic and sensory fibers. Injury to the nerve may be the cause of this short circuiting. Also, heat and algesic chemicals such as substance P, and bradykinin are thought to influence this crossover. Another vicious cycle is set up, which prolongs the pain and tenderness of RSD. What causes the ephase in RSD without a primary diagnosis, i.e., idiopathic, remains unanswered.

The final hypothesis to be considered concerns the gate control theory.[31] Melzak and Wall proposed that, under normal conditions, large afferent fibers (A beta) carrying proprioception, pressure, and light touch act to inhibit small diameter pain fibers (A delta and C). This control occurs in the substantia gelatinosa of the spinal cord. When large fibers "close the gate" to small fiber stimulation, the impulse is prohibited transmission through the dorsal horn to the cortex, and pain is not perceived. Research has disagreed with some of the gate control theory; evidence has been produced that small fibers also act as a presynaptic inhibitor, as do large fibers.[30] Sunderland[29] states that a breakdown in the control does not explain the RSD pain which follows complete injuries such as avulsion of cervical roots and nerve transections. Also, the spontaneous pain experienced without external stimuli is questioned. Those who believe that large fiber stimulation closes the gate to pain use treatments such as transcutaneous nerve stimulation or bombarding the system with numerous sensory provoking modalities, in order to override the pain impulse.

Anatomy

Treatment techniques for RSD and RP are developed as man's knowledge in neuropathology and anatomy grows. Just recently, the sympathetic fibers have been microscopically localized in the hand. Using fluorescent staining, the sympathetic fibers were identified at the peripheral edge of the median and ulnar epineurium and were not seen within the central portion of any nerve.[32] Staining of digital arteries revealed that the sympathetics are limited to the adventitia. This experimental technique substantiated the assumption that sympathetic fibers accompany major peripheral nerves and divide to supply arterial innervation. When sympathetic impulses reach the neuroeffector junctions in the adventitia of vessels, the catecholamine norepinephrine is released from granular sacs.[33] This neurotransmitter reacts with the alpha receptor to cause vasoconstriction of the vessel. Sympathetic stimulation also initiates a response in the sweat gland; here the fibers are cholinergic, emitting the transmitter acetylcholine. Ducts of these sweat glands open onto the papillary ridges, releasing a sodium chloride solution. The proximal component of these efferent sympathetic fibers is as complex as a road map.

From its cell body in the mediolateral column of the thoracic and upper lumbar spinal cord, the fiber exits from the cord through the ventral horn.[33,34] Once outside, the preganglionic sympathetic fiber divides from the cerebrospinal fiber and travels a short distance as a white communicating ramus. This leads to a paravertebral ganglion, which houses a neuron and the site for synapse between the preganglionic and postganglionic fiber. From the ganglion, the gray communicating ramus supplies the route for the sympathetic fiber to again join the spinal nerve. Paravertebral ganglions are located in each side of the vertebral column, from the upper cervical to the sacral area and are interconnected to form chains.

In the cervical region, there are three ganglia in each chain. The largest and most inferior, the stellate ganglion, is located between the transverse process of C-8 and the common carotid artery. Frequently it is joined with the first thoracic ganglion. Blocking sympathetic impulses from this site not only causes upper extremity vasodilatation and hypohydrosis, but also homolateral facial changes, i.e., Horner's syndrome. A contracted pupil due to paralysis of the iridodilator fibers and ptosis of the upperlid, a result of smooth muscle paralysis, are expected.[35]

CLINICAL MANIFESTATIONS OF RP

The prolonged and exaggerated cold response of those with Raynaud's phenomenon causes the following intermittent skin discolorations: (1) pallor due to a decrease in blood flow to the capillaries, (2) cyanosis caused by sluggish blood flow in dilated capillaries and venules, and lastly (3) rubor, the result of reactive hyperemia.[36] Pain[37] and a decrease in functional ability[38,39] often accompany these changes in blood flow. It has been documented that during short-term cold exposure, the reduction in finger dexterity and the pain perception of those with RP is statistically greater than that of a group of controls.[40] Also, the time required for the digital temperature of a cold extremity to return to its baseline, or resting temperature, is prolonged. Some authors report that those with RP require 30 minutes of re-warming time, compared to the normal of 5 to 10 minutes.[41] Diminished sensibility has also been suggested as a plight of Raynaud's subjects,[42] but this parameter requires further scrutiny.

Primary RP usually affects women in their early 20s.[6] As noted previously, the condition should be bilateral and symmetrical, i.e., all digits exhibit the phenomenon with equal intensity. Gangrenous digits are rare in primary RP. When the condition presents itself unilaterally, the possibility of thoracic outlet syndrome, cold injury, vibration, or drug-induced symptoms should be questioned. Most likely, secondary RP is the correct diagnosis.

Evaluation of RP

Diagnosing the patient may not be the primary concern of the physical therapist, but a thorough evaluation and understanding of the test results can only ensure proper patient care. Thulesius outlined a method for evaluation of patients with suspected RP.[43] Physical examination includes the Allen's test for patency of the radial and ulnar arteries, palpation of pulses for possible arterial obstruction, and auscultation of the subclavian artery for bruits and indications of stenosis or compression. Questioning the patient should include (1) occupation; use of vibratory tools or prolonged exposure to cold such as fish packing[44] or butchering, (2) smoking habits; decrease in blood flow[45] to the hands is associated with thromboangiitis obliterans, and (3) contact with certain chemicals, ergot, methysergide, and heavy metals, since all of the above can cause secondary RP. Next, the appearance of the patient's face and hands should be noted. Protruding fingernails and pulp atrophy are as typical to someone with scleroderma as are inelastic facial skin and a smooth tight mouth.

A subjective statement of ulnar parathesia, weakness of the arm, and typical RP may indicate arterial compression at the thoracic outlet. Adson, costoclavicular, and hyperabduction tests are sometimes helpful in a differential diagnosis. X-ray for cervical rib identification, nerve conduction velocity, and Doppler readings during the upper extremity maneuvers are recommended, if the diagnosis is not clear.[46] X-rays also assist in the diagnosis of RA and, if calcification of the pulp is exhibited, scleroderma is suggested. Barium studies help to confirm this diagnosis. Arteriography identifies blocked vessels and is most useful in the diagnosis of thromboembolisms due to thoracic outlet syndromes.[5] A less invasive technique, plethysmography, measures systolic blood pressure and verifies a clinical diagnosis of stenosis or occlusion. Pulse wave formation can identify vasospastic abnormalities and occlusive arterial disease.[43] Recently, radial isotope imaging has been used to assess distal circulation.[44] Laboratory tests can assist with the diagnosis of connective tissue disease and the presence of cold agglutinins and cryoglobulin. If no contributing factors can be identified, a diagnosis of primary RP is given.

RSD

Signs and symptoms of RSD vary as the patient progresses through three phases of the syndrome.[27,48] Pain is the common denominator for all stages and all patients, whereas, the degree of bone, skin, blood vessel, and muscle involvement differs. The confusing and endless terminology already described may be the result of patients' exhibiting varying manifestations.

Stage 1

Stage 1 may begin immediately or several weeks after trauma. This stage is characterized by a burning or aching type of pain, which is aggravated by attempted motion or by emotional stress. The initial vasodilatation will cause extensive and, often, pitting edema. A warm, erythemic, dry hand will develop coolness, cyanosis, and sweating due to altered vasomotor activity. Swelling persists as blood is trapped in the venous system. This pooling of fluid, especially over the dorsum of the hand, is due to the lack of upper extremity motion. Moberg described the necessity of a muscular pumping action to propel venous and lymphatic contents.[49]

Towards the end of this phase, which lasts for 3 to 6 months, radiographic changes develop. Bone density depletion has been documented as early as 38 and 40 days after onset.[50] Kozin et al., theorized that an increase in blood flow is responsible for the "patch" demineralization that they and Genant et al.[51] reported. This appearance, they state, is due to irregular reabsorption of trabecular bone. In addition to describing five patterns of osteoporotic changes, three patterns of erosive disease were identified. Surface erosions were characteristically similar to early RA changes. When using fine-detail roentgenography, significant diffuse and articular soft tissue swellings were identified.

In another study by Kozin et al.,[52] the histologic appearance of synovial biopsies was reported. There was an increase in the number of blood vessels proliferated, and unorganized synovial living cells were identified. Loose areolar connective tissue of the synovium was fibrosed. Also assessed were dolorimeter scores, which measure the degree of tenderness. These were significantly greater over articular regions, as compared to interarticular areas.

Stage 2

Prolonged vasomotor instability leads to the characteristic changes found in Stage 2. Brawny edema and joint contractures develop during this stage, which lasts from 3 to 6 months. The excessive tissue fluid of pitting edema is the perfect environment for the deposition of collagen fibers, which lead to brawny edema.[53] Pain remains constant but changes in character to become more pressure-like. Pain and edema both contribute to decreased mobility and eventual joint contractures. Shortening of the joint connective tissues may be due to the formation of new collagen[54] or the increase in the number of intermolecular crosslinks.[55] Peacock theorized that collagen was being synthesized, because of increased hydroxyproline content he measured in canine extremities after these joints were immobilized for 4 weeks.[54] The volar capsule was cited as the tissue responsible for the flexion contracture. Another researcher, using rat models, suggested that an increase in the quantity of reducible intermolecular cross-links was the cause of joint contracture.[55] Immobilization with a resultant decrease in water and proteoglycans is theorized to allow cross-linking at intercepts points and to allow random fiber orientation. Accompanying decreases in mobility and joint contracture is decreased muscle length due to a reduction in sarcomere.[56] How the epimysium is affected by immobilization has not yet been reported.

Other findings during stage 2 include skin and trophic alterations. Smooth shiny skin, muscle atrophy, Dupuytren-like contractures, and brittle grooved fingernails describe the outward changes. The unseen pathology of the bone and joint, already described in stage 1, continues or intensifies.

Stage 3

When stage 3 is reached, osteoporosis is diffuse and marked. Edema subsides, the remaining enlargement being periarticular. Typically, the more distal joints have the greatest degree of joint limitation. Joint contractures of stage 2 can develop into ankylosis. Atrophied fat pads, skin, and muscle, especially the interosseous, are evident. As the blood flow diminishes, skin temperature decreases, and the skin appearance remains glistening, with the loss of creases and wrinkles. Due to trophic changes, the fingers become pointed and thin with rigid nails. Eventually nail and hair growth may return to normal, and pain may be exacerbated only during attempted motions. The other possibility is that the pain will last for years and become intractable.

RSD Personality Manifestation

A result of this prolonged pain may be an alteration in personality.[57] Initially a manic state may be demonstrated, then the patient becomes withdrawn. A characteristic exhibited by six RSD patients on a Life Goal Inventory assessment was their "willingness to assume hardship."[58] Using the MMPI, Subbarao[59] found that 32 of his 45 patients showed hysteria and hypochondriasis, while 28 were depressed. Hardy[60] compared patients with hand injuries to those with RSD and found a significant difference in: body cathexis, interpersonal sensitivity, somatization, depression, and anxiety. It has been suggested that not only do these traits heighten and lengthen the syndrome, but they also predispose a person to this disability.

RSD MANAGEMENT

The age old adage,"Don't put off till tomorrow, what you can do today," has merit when considering the treatment of RSD. Early recognition and management affords good results; whereas, the consequence of delayed treatment may be only satisfactory, although the management is more involved. When treating those with the initial symptoms of RSD, Kleinert[61] used physical therapy and mood modifying medications. This was the only treatment necessary to allow patients full functioning without pain. The patients who exhibited advanced signs received stellate ganglion blocks; of the 183 patients, two-thirds had permanent improvement, and 23 patients underwent sympathectomies, 19 experiencing good results. Poplawski and colleagues[62] managed their 28 RSD patients with lidocaine, corticosteroids, and physical therapy. They reported poor results in seven cases where patients had developed RSD at least 9 months prior to treatment; all other patients had good to excellent results.

Often the therapist treating the patients with Colles fracture or CVA will be the one most likely to identify the developing symptoms of pain, edema, and discoloration. It is the therapist's responsibility to notify the physician of his other concern, to begin accurate recording of baseline measurements, and to initiate immediate treatment. Prior to beginning any treatment, baseline digital temperature, active range of motion, pain perception, and volumetric measurement should be recorded.

Baseline Measurement for Treatment

Room temperature should be constant for all finger temperature recordings. The patient should sit in a position of comfort, maintaining one hand position, and the digital temperature should be recorded when the temperature has oscillated no more than $0.2°C$ within 4 minutes[63]. Pain perception can be assessed by the use of a 10 cm horizontal visual analog scale.[64]

| Pain as bad as it could be | |————————————————————| | No pain |

A standard explanation of the scale should be given, but a number value should not be suggested. The patient estimates his pain perception by placing a vertical line on the scale, and the therapist records a ± 0.5 cm value in the patient's chart. To establish a baseline value of edema, circumferential or volumetric measurements can be used. Once baseline values are recorded, treatment may begin. Reevaluation may be carried out when necessary.

Treatment

Since pain, edema, and the lack of active use of the extremity are the components leading to a nonfunctional extremity, these must be addressed immediately. Pain halts active motion which assists in edema reduction, and therefore pain control should receive top priority. Therapeutic modalities such as heat and cold, intravenous injections, stellate ganglion block, transcutaneous nerve stimulation (TENS), and sympathectomy have all been used to decrease pain. Therapists can directly administer several of the above and should be involved in monitoring the patient's active exercise which follows all treatments.

Using prolonged heat or cold was found successful in the treatment of 53 out of 63 patients, as reported by Johnson and Pannozzo.[65] Continuous paraffin baths for 6 to 7 hours were interrupted by periods of active exercise. Other authors have used ultrasound, short wave, microwave, infrared, contrast baths, ice packs, and whirlpool in an attempt to bombard the system with sensory stimuli and, thereby, to decrease pain. Of the patients utilizing several modalities, paraffin and contrast baths were considered to afford the greatest relief of symptoms.[59]

When Omar and Thomas[66] used only physical modalities to treat their 41 patients, 9 improved. Less than one-third of their patients had symptoms for over 6 weeks. Because most of the literature lacks documentation of modalities received, length of treatment time, and whether additional therapeutic procedures were given, interpreting the results is difficult, and the therapist is left to rely on his or her own experience. Bombarding the system with physical modalities is successful for some patients, but not for all.

Ultrasound, cited as a thermal modality, has also been used directly over the stellate ganglion for its analgestic effects.[67] Daily, pulsed ultrasound at 1 to 1.5 watts/cm^2 for 7 to 8 minutes was used in conjunction with other modalities. Goodman reports that six out of seven patients perceived a decrease in pain. Pain relief was evident in one case in 15 days and in another patient 1 month after treatment was initiated. Suggested advantages of this technique over surgery and procaine injection are that it is reversible, a Horner's syndrome is not produced, and a foreign substance is not injected into the body. The effects of ultrasound on the ganglion are not broached by the author.

Another form of pain control, TENS, seems similar, in theory, to stimuli bombardment, as both methods activate large A-alpha and beta fibers. Conventional TENS units are set for a high pulse rate (50 to 100 Hz) and a narrow pulse width (45 to 75 μ seconds).[68] Amplitude is monitored so that paresthesia is perceived and no muscle contraction is evident. Electrode placement is over the peripheral nerve proximal to the site of injury.[69] Relief of pain may be dramatic or adequate to allow a simultaneous therapy program of exercise. In addition to surface electrodes, needle electrodes have been used to quiet intractable pain. This treatment affords a numb and painfree extremity for approximately half an hour.[70]

Conservative management of pain includes the use of connective tissue massage. It is claimed that when applied two to three times daily for 20 minutes, the effect is complete pain relief. Whether this technique succeeds because it acts as a counter-irritant, or causes enkephalin release is unknown.[71] Only one case report utilizes this treatment technique.

Steroid Management

What necessitates the progression from conservative hand therapy to the use of corticosteroids or blocks is determined individually. Some authors utilize them immediately, whereas others wait for the initial results of therapy. Persistent and relentless pain and edema signify lack of treatment effectiveness and the need for alternate or additional measures. When comparing corticosteroid treatment to other steroid anti-inflammatory drugs, beta and alpha blockers, and stellate block, six subjects treated with steroids had uniformly beneficial responses.[52] They had statistically significant decrements in joint tenderness and swelling. Prednisone was given daily for up to 2 weeks and then every other day. A disadvantage to this treatment was worsening of symptoms as the dosage was lowered or halted. In another study of 17 patients undergoing prednisone treatment, 82 ranked their pain relief as good or excellent, whereas the 7 who received stellate blocks considered their pain relief fair or poor.[50]

Procaine Management

Reduction in pain by injecting procaine or lidocaine has been successful in some cases. Injecting lidocaine and methylprednisolone intravenously allowed painfree passive exercise in Poplawski's group of RSD patients. During the 30-minute treatment session, controlled mobilization, deep friction massage, and passive stretching was performed.[62] Following the nerve block, therapy continued and included active exercise. Most patients required two to three blocks and some needed five. Criteria for subsequent blocks were return of pain and stiffness, loss of motion, and plateauing of progress. Sixteen of the 28 patients considered their results good or better. Good was defined as the rare occurrence of discomfort, and some stiffness. As already noted, the seven patients who had had symptoms for 9 months or longer had poor results.

Management of Sympathectomy Blocks

If a localized area of pain can be identified, peripheral infusion sympathectomy may be considered. Into a trigger point, an area of extreme irritation, is inserted an intravenous catheter. Lidocaine is periodically injected through the catheter. Again, active exercise is performed when the extremity is pain-free. When this technique was used for seven patients, five considered themselves improved.[66] Injections frequently averaged 2.2 hours when the patient was in stage 1, and lengthened as pain decreased. This treatment was not recommended for those with brachial plexus injuries or those with pain in the contralateral, unaffected extremity, or for those with pain lasting longer than 3 months. Again, delayed treatment equals poor results.

Diminished pain or pain-free exercise can be accomplished after stellate ganglion blocks. A successful block is one that affords an immediate decrease in pain, an increase in skin temperature, a Horner's syndrome, and a delayed reduction in edema. These can be measured pre- and post-block to evaluate the effectiveness of the block. Evaluation by thermograms and psychogalvanic reflex also assists in assessing the interruption of sympathetic impulses. The number of blocks performed and the interim period vary according to the patient's needs and the physician in charge. Daily blocks for 7 days are not unusual; as many as 14 blocks have been administered. With each additional block, the duration of subsequent pain relief should increase. If three or four blocks do not decrease pain, the treatment should be discontinued.

Sympathetic Management

If immediate but not prolonged pain relief results from a course of sympathetic blocks, sympathectomy may be considered. In a study of 31 surgical sympathectomy patients, 20 cases had good to excellent pain relief and all had decreased cyanosis and increased sweating.[73] Those with symptoms of prolonged duration, the average being approximately 35 months, had poor results. Other researchers have found that those in stage 3 do not respond as well to sympathectomy.

Temperature Biofeedback Management

Relief of pain by obliterating sympathetic control is dramatic, when considering the permanent effects of surgical sympathectomy. To control these impulses rather than totally to sever their influence would benefit the patient. Autonomic control such as temperature biofeedback could assist these patients to gain this vasomotor regulation. Detailed discussion of this treatment modality will be presented in the section on management of RP.

While attempts are being made to decrease pain, concurrent efforts are established to reduce edema and maintain range of motion. During pain-free intervals, active range of motion and functional activities should be encouraged. Since pain management is the primary concern, the exercise program should not aggravate the condition; rather, motions should take place within the comfort range. Treatment should make the most of the pain-free time, and sessions 3 hours long are not uncommon.

As the patient progresses, the treatment regime, functional activities, and the home program should become more demanding, but not increased in complexity, as it has been suggested that this group of patients requires a structured and simplistic program.[58]

Edema control can take many avenues, and not all methods are tolerated well by every patient. Elevation, retrograde massage, Isotoner* and Jobst† gloves, airsplints, Jobst† intermittent compression, and high volt galvanic stimulation are a few ways to assist in edema reduction. Active motion, as Moberg stated, is a key to maintaining normal circulation. Successful use of the hand as a pump depends on unlimited range of motion and a strong contraction.

---

*Arisgloves, 417 5th Ave, New York, NY 10016
†Jobst Inc, Box 853, Toledo OH 43694.

Splinting

Often wrist stabilization is necessary to allow full use of the available finger range of motion. Splinting to achieve the above is acceptable. No increase in pain should result, and there must be unrestricted finger motion.

As the patient progresses, dynamic splinting may be required to increase finger flexion. MP cuffs with a wrist strap, PIP-DIP cuffs, or rubberband traction to the distal palmar crease may help to achieve the patient's goal of increased motion. Residual pain limited to one joint, such as the shoulder, may respond well to phonophoresis with Hydrocortisone cream, and capsular adhesions can be combatted with Iodex phonophoresis. Using iontophoresis for pain and adhesion reduction is also appropriate.

Summary

In summary, a therapist possesses many skills and modalities with which to treat the patient with RSD. Not all methods work equally well with all patients. Keystones of management should be pain control, edema reduction, and active range of motion. Early recognition and management will produce the best result. Patients with obvious psychological problems, whether they evolve around the disability or were present beforehand should be addressed.

The therapist's counseling skills can often decrease the patient's anxiety and give reassurance. Occasionally, the patient's psychological problems are beyond the realm of the therapist, and this must be recognized. A patient who realizes that psychiatric help is a routine therapy given to all patients with hand injuries may accept assistance without alarm. Not to offer a valuable therapy such as this for fear of rebuttal is an injustice to the patient. The patient is ready for discharge when his or her progress has plateaued and the therapist is satisfied that all beneficial methods of treatment have been explored. Periodic re-evaluations will reveal no increase in range of motion or functional level. Functional ability can be assessed subjectively or by a standardized test such as the Purdue pegboard and/or Moberg's pick-up test.

Prior to discharge, all patients should demonstrate the ability to carry out an independent home program. The possibility of relapse exists, and the therapist must relate to the patient that if symptoms recur, immediate medical attention should be sought. In some cases, a follow-up reevaluation scheduled for 1 or 3 months post-discharge is incentive for the patient to continue his or her home program, and it also allows the therapist an opportunity to identify recurrence.

CASE PRESENTATION

A 67-year-old white female sustained a Colles fracture to her right, dominant wrist. Included in her pertinent medical history is that 1 year prior to her fracture she was hospitalized for 1 month for neuritis that involved all four extremities.

While her wrist fracture was casted she complained that it was too tight, but waited for 2 weeks before seeking medical advice. When her cast was trimmed, extensive edema was noted about the thumb, and this was her area of greatest pain. Following this, she had no further distress or complaints about the cast. As the cast was removed, at 6 weeks post-injury, she became faint and had "excruciating pain." At this time, no edema was noted; she was fitted with a cock-up splint. Two days later she returned to the physician with marked dorsal edema, a cyanotic distal arm, and a painful right upper extremity.

Tylenol with Codeine was prescribed, and hand therapy was begun. Daily 3-hour therapy sessions for 5 days did not decrease the patient's pain perception, or her edema, nor increase her active range of motion. Treatment consisted of local ice to the shoulder, whirlpool at 96°F massage, elevated loom activities, and other active exercises. Although TENS was demonstrated on the therapist and then on the patient's unaffected extremity, she became very anxious and apprehensive about its use on the right arm. Because of this, TENS was not used, and the benefits, if any, were not appreciated. Heat, isotoner gloves, and airsplints aggravated the patient in this stage of RSD. She had restless nights and a constant headache. She openly discussed her pain with all other hand patients. Continual verbal reassurance and praise were given during her therapy treatments.

Because of the lack of progress, the physician was notified, and a joint decision made to hospitalize the patient for daily stellate ganglion blocks and intensive therapy twice daily. During her week of hospitalization, she successfully received four Marcaine blocks. Each block afforded her diminished pain, and daily improvement in all phases of therapy was documented. She tolerated pendulum exercises and found that a 2-pound weight around the wrist improved her motion. This patient achieved the greatest range of motion when the therapist allowed her to perform her exercises independently. This was true because the patient feared forceful, painful motions and enjoyed controlling her own program. Cold whirlpools with the patient squeezing a sponge cylinder, massage, and ice were continued and were effective in decreasing her edema for short periods of time.

She was asked to increase her involvement in functional activities, beginning with ADLs. Washing, dressing, and feeding were practiced; this patient required constant reminders to utilize the right upper extremity. Built-up utensil handles were supplied to allow eating with the right, dominant hand. Periarticular swelling was evident around the IP joints. These joints and the shoulder were the sites of concentrated pain. Grade 2 mobilization for these joints was tolerated well.

At hospital discharge, the home program was reviewed. Again, Tylenol with Codeine was given. Daily therapy sessions continued, and a plateau was again reached 3 weeks after hospital discharge. The patient had 140° of shoulder flexion, full internal rotation, 45° of external rotation, and 120° of shoulder abduction. A painful shoulder was limiting further improvement in the patient's daily activities for therapy. A sudden movement of the shoulder would elicit pain, and occasionally, without reason, a knife-stabbing type of pain was perceived. Trigger point injection of procaine into the upper trapezium resulted in improved shoulder range of motion over the next week of therapy and decreased pain. The patient was then able to assist her daughter, who owned a restaurant-bar. Folding laundry and washing dishes were done with little immediate discomfort, but unless the patient rested following these activities, edema and cyanosis resulted. Light resistive exercises using a weight well caused no discomfort.

Although pain perception had significantly diminished since her initial visit, pain and occasional hand edema were still limiting total rehabilitation. Medrol, a corticosteroid, was prescribed in a 5-day pack. Since taking this drug, the patient has had no hand edema. On cold days her right hand appears cyanotic and feels cooler to her. She has occasional shoulder pain, and her active range of motion is 165° of shoulder flexion, full internal rotation, 150° of abduction, and 60° of external rotation. Passively her finger tips touch the distal palmar crease; actively she lacks ½ cm. Her thumb continues to have a "strange feeling" similar to that experienced when she had neuritis. At the time of this writing, the patient is seen twice weekly for a strengthening program.

RP MANAGEMENT EVALUATION

The purpose of the pretreatment evaluation for those with RP is two-fold. First, the diagnosis of primary or secondary RP must be discerned, and, secondly, baseline objective and subjective measurements must be recorded. These parameters will be reevaluated following the completion of the treatments. Procedures recommended for this physical examination have already been discussed. If the therapist thinks further laboratory or x-ray studies need to be completed, these should be recommended to the physician.

Baseline evaluation should include documentation of resting finger temperature and a test of finger dexterity and pain perception after cold exposure. The cold stimulus can be presented in one of two ways and is dependent on the type of equipment available. If a flat disc tele-thermometer is at hand, the thermister can be taped to a middle finger and the hand covered with a plastic glove. This hand is lowered into ice water and remains there until the skin temperature reaches 13°C. When the disc-type thermister is not available, a constant length of cold water immersion is used instead of the constant finger temperature being reached. Twenty seconds of the ice water bath has been recommended.[10]

Pain perception can be evaluated on the scale previously described. Finger dexterity has been tested by using a right-handed Purdue test, and was also evaluated before the cold stimulus was presented.[40] If the Purdue test is not available, another similar functional test may be substituted, such as the O'Conner test. Room temperature must be constant, the cold stimulus and also the pain scale must be presented in the same fashion, and the functional test must remain constant from evaluation to evaluation.

In addition to the above tests, the therapist may evaluate the time necessary for the finger temperature to return to baseline following cold exposure. Also, the sensibility of the patient after the cold stimulus may be assessed. When two point discrimination was evaluated before and after the cold stimulus, no statistical difference was found between a control and a Raynaud's group.[40] Another sensory instrument may document the diminished sensibility that patents have described. All of the above evaluations may be necessary to objectively identify patient improvement, but due to the type of treatment or the equipment available, only some tests will need to be completed. In the past, subjective measurements have been used to report the success of treatments. Future, objective evaluations will provide validity to the treatment techniques.

Management—Short-Term Techniques

Management of Raynaud's patients can be divided into two groups—treatments that afford palliative temporary relief and treatments with more permanent long-lasting effects. Short-term techniques include rapidly swinging the arms in large circles, so that gravitational and centrifugal forces assist in blood flow,[73] and wearing electrically heated gloves[74] or hand warmers similar to those used by hunters. TENS has also been cited for its value in the treatment of RP. Kaada, as described by Mannheimer,[68] was able to produce vasodilatation and increased skin temperature when a 2 Hz burst rate was used, 0.2 ms pulse duration, and 20 to 30 ms intensity. A 30- to 45-minute treatment session yielded relief of symptoms for 4 to 8 hours.

Management—Long-Term Techniques

The following techniques are considered long-term since, once the techniques have been learned, the benefits are reaped for months to years, although the patient may require occasional reinstruction in the technique. Classical conditioning has allowed vasodilatation in primary Raynaud's patients. Pairing whole body exposure to cold (0°C) and hands to warm water (43°C) resulted in a learned response.[75] Three times weekly for 3 weeks, each patient warmed their hands in 49°C water (or air). They then sat for 10 minutes in a cold chamber, while keeping their hands in warm water. After these treatment sessions, they were able to maintain their digital temperature at a significantly higher temperature during cold exposure. These effects were evaluated 4 months post-treatment, and the digital temperature remained higher than the pretreatment measurement. In the past, alteration in digital temperature and blood flow has been achieved by autogenic training. This technique can consist of vivid imagery, "I'm lying on a hot, sandy beach," or suggestive phrases such as "my hands are heavy and warm," or hypnotic suggestions or relaxation exercises. A therapist may choose the above method of treatment or another form of self-regulation, temperature biofeedback. It has been suggested that controlling the sympathetics through this technique involves the hypothalamus and limbic system. Altering the autonomic system may be difficult because of the factors outlined by Taub.[76] First, sensory inflow from the vascular system is over small diameter unmyelinated fibers, and therefore, slow. Second, cortical representation is scant.

TEMPERATURE BIOFEEDBACK EVALUATION

Various methods for teaching temperature regulation have been used, and often a combination of imagery and biofeedback is taught. Generally, auditory and visual feedback supplies the patient with immediate knowledge of his or her success or failure at temperature control. Some authors place one thermister on the forehead and one on the fingertip and ask the patient to increase the hand temperature above the forehead temperature; others monitor just the finger temperature. Until recently, patients were not given cold stress tests, and the merit of biofeedback was based upon a decrease in the frequency and severity of the attacks. This subjective information is valuable, and the patient may keep a record of this while learning self regulation. Gerber found that, following biofeedback training, both primary and secondary Raynaud's patients were able to maintain a higher finger temperature during cold exposure.[77] Surwit also documented that primary Raynaud's patients would significantly improve their cold stress temperature by practicing autogenic training.[78] Slide projections and taped suggestions are thought to enhance digital control, but how long imagery remains valuable is questioned.[79] A copy of the researchers' slide-suggestion combination is available by writing to Edward Taub, Institute of Behavioral Research, 2429 Linden Lane, Silver Spring, Maryland, 20910.

A cold environment causes decreased finger dexterity, strength, and sensibility in normals.[80] When a group of controls was instructed in temperature regulation by the use of imagery, classical conditioning, and temperature biofeedback, they were able to perform in a cold chamber without a significant decrement in any of the above paramenters. Cold stressing and evaluating the Raynaud's patient who is proficient in temperature regulation could objectively assess this treatment. Future research in this area needs to be completed.

Temperature Biofeedback Techniques

To learn temperature control, the normal subjects practice in a warm climate prior to cold exposure. The following treatment continuum of increased diversion and cold exposure may teach the Raynaud's patient to maintain temperature regulation: (1) the patient sits in a quiet, temperature-controlled room and practices imagery or biofeedback; (2) a cold stimulus such as a glass of ice water is touched, and the patient is asked to maintain the warm finger temperature; (3) small objects such as nuts and bolts are placed in cold water, and the patient is asked to interlock them, while temperature control is practiced; and (4) the patient repeats the first three steps while seated in a busy clinic.

Most patients want to avoid a Raynaud's attack while they carry out daily activities, such as reaching in the refrigerator, mixing meatloaf, and drinking ice tea. The above treatment program should allow them to function at that level. If the patient desires digital control while the total body is exposed to cold, more extensive training will be needed. It is unknown whether a Raynaud's patient can gain such control.

PATIENT EDUCATION

Educating the patient is an invaluable part of the therapy. An explanation of the patient's condition may be all the therapy necessary. For example, a farmer with primary Raynaud's phenomenon was referred for temperature biofeedback. He was confused about his condition and troubled because he lacked control of this phenomenon. Following a basic anatomy lesson and presentation to him of the theories of RP, he was instructed in temperature biofeedback. He rented a thermister for home practice, only to return it in 1 week, stating that he knew how to regulate his temperature and was relieved that this problem was so insignificant.

Home programs are generally given, and temperature sensitive tapes, small battery operated digital thermometers, or hand-held thermometers can be issued to assist in temperature feedback. Teaching a patient to regulate his temperature may require only four 1-hour sessions or could necessitate months of practice. If the therapist does not consider self-regulation a viable treatment for RP, this attitude will be perceived by the patient, and the treatment will be a failure. A therapist with the above attitude would teach only 2 out of 22 subjects to control their temperature, whereas, a person who believes in the feasibility of the treatment can teach 19 out of 21.[76]

DRUG MANAGEMENT

Drug management for Raynaud's phenomenon is aimed at either reducing sympathetic tone or improving the blood flow properties. As with temperature self-regulation techniques, the success of drug management stands on the patient's report of decreased frequency and severity of attacks, improvement in cold recovery time, and the healing of digital ulcers. By performing objective evaluations prior to and following drug therapy, the therapist can assist the physician in recognizing a beneficial treatment. Also, the therapist should be aware of the common drug side effects, such as drowsiness, fluid retention, weight gain, weakness, depression, orthostatic hypotension, and tachycardia.

SURGICAL MANAGEMENT

Surgical management includes vein graphs for thrombosed radial or ulnar arteries,[47] digital artery sympathectomy,[22] or axillary sympathectomy. Digital artery sympathectomy has decreased pain and increased digital temperature for patients with Raynaud's phenomenon; as with the other treatments, no objective evaluation of functional ability has been performed. With the reported success of digital sympathectomies, the more proximal sympathectomy will probably become infrequent.

SUMMARY

The literature to date does not use large samples of primary RP subjects and secondary RP subjects for comparison. Which of the above techniques are effective for one and not the other is generally unknown. Not all people with RP require treatment; some people may stop using vibratory tools and have a remission of symptoms. Others may quit smoking, and still others, when educated about the effects of emotional stress, may need no further treatment. Conservative management should be exhausted prior to surgical intervention.

CONCLUSIONS

Raynaud's phenomenon and reflex sympathetic dystrophy syndrome are the results of vasomotor disturbances. Pain, the primary symptom, affects the patient suffering from either diagnosis. In order to control their pain, patients with RSD may require months of therapy, in conjunction with other medical treatments. Even then, the results may be devastating, i.e., a nonfunctional upper extremity with intractable pain. If the patient is treated when the symptoms are first noted, good results may prevail.

Bombarding the patient with sensory stimuli such as heat, cold, and TENS has been effective in decreasing the RSD patient's pain. Corticosteroids and drug blocks may be necessary to further diminish their pain. Hopefully, sympathectomy is not required. Temperature biofeedback or a similar technique of self-regulation may assist the RSD patient in vasomotor control, as it does the patient with Raynaud's phenomenon. Eradicating sympathetic tone at the digital arteries is a fairly new and successful treatment for RP.

Both types of patients require psychological support and understanding of their conditions. In the case of the patient with RP, this may be all the treatment required, and, in the patient with RSD, perhaps more professional help may be needed.

To advance our treatment regimes, thorough evaluation and documentation must begin in the clinic. From there, research is born, which feeds our professional growth and benefits our patients.

REFERENCES

1. Drucker W, Hubay C, Holden W, Bukovnic J: Pathogenesis of post-traumatic sympathetic dystrophy. Am J Surg 97:454, 1959
2. Peacock J: Peripheral venous blood concentrations of epinephrine and norepinephrine in primary Raynaud's disease. Circ Res 7:821, 1959
3. Kosin F, Ryan L, Carerra G et al: The reflex sympathetic dystrophy syndrome. Am J Med 70:23, 1981
4. Allen E, Brown G: Raynaud's disease: A critical review of minimal requisites for diagnosis. Am J Med Sci 183:187, 1932
5. Birnstingl M: The Raynaud syndrome. Postgrad Med J 47:297, 1971
6. Thulesius O: Primary and secondary Raynaud phenomena. Acta Chir Scand (Suppl.) 465: 5, 1976
7. Graham D: Cutaneous vascular reactions in Raynaud's disease and in states of hostility, anxiety and depression. Psychosom Med 17:200, 1955
8. Mittelmann B, Wolff H: Affective states and skin temperature: Experimental study of subjects with "cold hands" and Raynaud's syndrome. Psychosom Med 1(2):271, 1939
9. Folkow B, Fox R, Krog J et al: Studies on the reactions of the cutaneous vessels to cold exposure. Acta Physiol Scand 58:342, 1963
10. Porter J, Bardana E, Baur G et al: The clinical significance of Raynaud's syndrome. Surgery 80:756, 1976
11. Dabich L, Bookstein J, Zweifler A, Zarafonetis C: Digital arteries in patients with scleroderma. Arch Intern Med 130:708, 1972
12. Norton W: Comparison of the microangiopathy of systemic lupus erythematosus, dermatomyositis, scleroderma and diabetes mellitus. Lab Invest 22:301, 1970

13. Scott J, Hourihane D, Doyle F, Steiner R et al: Digital arteritis in rheumatoid disease. Ann Rheum Dis 20:224, 1961
14. Ashe W, Cook W, Old J: Raynaud's phenomenon of occupational origin. Arch Environ Health 5:333 1962
15. Pyykko R, Hyvarinen J: Vibration induced changes of sympathetic vasomotor tone. Acta Chir Scand, suppl. 465:23, 1976
16. Olesen H: The cold agglutinin syndrome. Dan Med Bull 14:138, 1967
17. Ritzmann S, Levin W: Cryopathies: A review. Rev Intern Med 107:754, 1961
18. Johnston E, Summerly R, Birnstingl M: Prognosis in Raynaud's phenomenon after sympatheclony. Br Med J 10:962, 1965
19. Ehrly A: Treatment of patients with secondary Raynaud's syndrome. Acta Chir Scand, suppl. 465:92, 1976
20. Jarrett P, Morland M, Browse N: Treatment of Raynaud's phenomenon by fibrinolytic enhancement. Br Med J 2:523, 1978
21. Simpson S, Brown G, Adson A: Raynaud's disease: evidence that it is a type of vasomotor neurosis. Arch Neurol Psychol 26(4):687, 1931
22. Flatt A: Digital artery sympathectomy. J Hand Surg 5:550, 1980
23. Peacock J: The effect of changes in local temperature on the blood flows of the normal hand, primary Raynaud's disease and primary acrocyanosis. Clin Sci 19:505, 1960
24. Hillestad L: Blood flow in vascular disorders: A plethysmographic study. Acta Med Scand 188:185, 1970
25. Nielsen S, Noben B, Hirai M, Eklof B: Raynaud's phenomenon in arterial obstructive disease of the hand demonstrated by locally provoked cooling. Scand J Thorac Cardiovasc Surg 12:105, 1978
26. Downey J, LeRoy E, Miller J, Darling R: Thermo regulation and Raynaud's phenomenon. Clin Sci 40:211, 1971
27. Steinbrocker O, Spitzer N, Friedman H: The shoulder-hand syndrome in reflex dystrophy of the upper extremity. Ann Intern Med 29:22, 1947
28. Steinbrocker O, Argyros T: The shoulder-hand syndrome: present status as a diagnostic and therapeutic entity. Arch Phys Med Rehabil 49:1533 1968
29. Sunderland S: Pain mechanisms in causalgia. J Neurol Neurosurg Psychiatry 39:471, 1976
30. Zimmerman M: Peripheral and central nervous mechanisms of nociception, pain and pain therapy: Facts and hypotheses. Adv Pain Res Ther 3:3, 1979
31. Melzack R, Wall P: Pain mechanisms: A new theory. Science 150:971, 1965
32. Morgan R, Reisman N, Wilgis E: Anatomic localization of sympathetic nerves in the hand. J Hand Surg 8:283, 1983
33. Ham A, Cormack D (eds): Histology. JB Lippincott Co, Philadelphia, 1979
34. Gray H: Gray's Anatomy. Bounty Books, New York, 1978
35. Bannister R (ed): Brain's Clinical Neurology. 4th Ed. Oxford University Pr Inc, 1973
36. McGrath M, Penny R: The mechanisms of Raynaud's phenomenon: Part 1. Med J Aust 2:328, 1974
37. Surwit R: Biofeedback, a possible treatment of Raynaud's disease. Semin Psy 5:483, 1973
38. Adair J, Theobald D: Raynaud's phenomenon: Treatment of a severe case with biofeedback. J Indiana State Med Assoc 71:990, 1978
39. Blanchard E, Haynes M: Biofeedback treatment of a case of Raynaud's disease. J Behav Ther Exp Psychiatry 6:230, 1975
40. Delp H: Effects of brief cold exposure on finger dexterity and sensibility in subjects with Raynaud's phenomenon, unpublished Master's thesis, Virginia Commonwealth University, Medical College of Virginia, 1982
41. Porter J, Snider R, Bardana E et al: The diagnosis and treatment of Raynaud's phenomenon. Surgery 77:11, 1975

42. Carlson W, Samueloff S, Taylor W, Wasserman D: Instrumentation for measurement of sensory loss in the fingertips. J Occup Med 21(4):260, 1979
43. Thulesius O: Methods for the evaluation of peripheral vascular function in the upper extremities. Acta Chir Scand (Suppl.) 465:53, 1976
44. Mackiewicz F, Piskorz A: Raynaud's phenomenon following long-term repeated action of great differences of temperature. J Cardiovasc Surg 18(2):151, 1977
45. Ludbrook J, Vincent A, Walsh J: The effects of sham smoking and tobacco smoking on hand blood flow. Australian J Exp Biol Med Sci 52:285, 1974
46. Eklöf B: Vascular compression syndromes of the upper extremity. Acta Chir Scand (Suppl.) 465:74, 1976
47. Wilgis E: Evaluation and treatment of chronic digital ischemia. Ann Surg. 193:693, 1981
48. Bonica J: Causalgia and other reflex sympathetic dystrophies. Postgrad Med 53(6):143, 1973
49. Moberg E: The shoulder-hand-finger syndrome. Surg Clin North Am 40:367, 1960
50. Kozin F, Genant H, Bekerman C et al: The reflex sympathetic dystrophy syndrome 11. Roentgenographic and scintigraphic evidence of bilaterality and of periarticular accentuation. Am J Med 60:332, 1976
51. Genant H, Kozin F, Bekerman C et al: A comprehensive analysis using fine-detail radiography, photon absorptiometry, and bone and joint scintigraphy. Radiology 117:21, 1975
52. Kozin F, Genant H, Bekerman C et al: The reflex sympathetic dystrophy syndrome. Clinical and histologic studies: Evidence for bilaterality, response to corticosteroids and articular involvement. Am J Med 60:321, 1976
53. Absoe-Hansen G, Dyrbye M, Moltke E: Tissue edema a stimulus of connective tissue regeneration. J Invest Dermatol 32:505, 1959
54. Peacock E: Some biochemical and biophysical aspects of joint stiffness: Role of collagen synthesis as opposed to altered molecular bonding. Ann Surg 164:1, 1966
55. Akeson W, Mechanic G, Woo S, et al: Collagen cross-linking alterations in joint contractures: Changes in the reducible cross-links in periarticular connective tissue collagen after nine weeks of immobilization. Conn Tissue Res 5:15, 1977
56. Tabary J, Tabary C: Physiological and structure changes in the cat's soleus muscle due to immobilization at different lengths by plaster casts. J Physiol (London) 224:231, 1972
57. Omer G: Sensibility testing. In Omer G, Spinner M (eds): Management of Peripheral Nerve Problems WB Saunders, Philadelphia, 1980
58. Waylett J: Behavioral Patterns in reflex sympathetic dystrophy. In Hunter J, Schneider L, Mackin E, Bell J (eds): Rehabilitation of the Hand CV Mosby Co, St. Louis, 1978
59. Subbarao J, Stillwell G: Reflex sympathetic dystrophy syndrome of the upper extremity: Analysis of total outcome of management of 125 cases. Arch Phys Med Rehabil 62:549, 1981
60. Hardy J: Peripheral inputs to the central regulation for body temperature. In Itoh S, Ogata K, Yoshimura H (eds): Advances in Climatic Physiology Igaku-Shoin New York, 1972
61. Kleinert H, Wayne L, Kutz J et al: Post-traumatic sympathetic dystrophy. Orthop Clin North Amer 4:917, 1973
62. Poplawski Z, Wiley A, Murray J: Post-traumatic dystrophy of the extremities. J Bone Joint Surg 65-A:642, 1983
63. Sdorow L, Palladino J: Length of baseline and skin temperature training. Biofeedback Self Regul 4(3):289, 1979
64. Scott J, Huskisson E: Graphic representation of pain. Pain 2:175, 1976
65. Johnson E, Pannozzo A: Management of shoulder-hand syndrome. JAMA 195:108, 1966
66. Omer G, Thomas S: The management of chronic pain syndromes in the upper extremity. Clin Orthop 104:37, 1974

67. Goodman C: Treatment of shoulder-hand syndrome. NY State J Med 71:559, 1971
68. Mannheimer J: TENS as as adjunctive technique in hand rehabilitation. APTA Section on Hand Rehabilitation. Vol. 1. No 3, 1983
69. Meyer G, Fields H: Causalgia treated by selective large fibre stimulation of peripheral nerve. Brain 95:163, 1972
70. Wall P, Sweet W, Temporary abolition of pain in Man. Science 155:108, 1967
71. Frazier F: Persistent post-sympathetic pain treated by connective tissue massage. Physio-therapy 64:211, 1978
72. Toumey J: Occurence and management of reflex sympathetic dystrophy. J Bone Joint Surg 30A:883, 1948
73. McIntyre D: A maneuver to reverse Raynaud's phenomenon of the fingers. JAMA 240: 2760, 1978
74. Kempson G, Coggon D, Acheson E: Electrically heated gloves for intermittent digital is-chaemia. Br Med J 286:268, 1983
75. Jobe J, Sampson J, Roberts D, et al: Induced vasodilation as treatment for Raynaud's dis-ease. Ann Intern Med 97:706, 1982
76. Taub E: Self-regulation of human tissue temperature. In Schwartz G, Beatty J (eds): Bio-feedback Theory and Research. Academic Press, New York, 1977
77. Geber L: Biofeedback for patients with Raynaud's phenomenon. JAMA 242:509, 1979
78. Surwit R, Shapiro D, Feld J: Digital temperature, autoregulation and associated cardiovas-cular changes. Psychophysiology 13:242, 1976
79. Herzfeld G, Taub E: Effect of slide projections and tape-recorded suggestions on thermal biofeedback training. Biofeedback Self Regul 5(4):393, 1980
80. Hayduk A: Increasing hand efficiency at cold temperatures by training hand vasodilation with a classical conditioning-biofeedback overlap design. Biofeedback Self Regul 5(3): 307, 1980

5 | Replantation: Current Clinical Treatment

Ellen Ring Horovitz
Patricia Theiss Casler

Successful replantation dates to 1962, when Malt replanted the arm of a 12-year-old boy.[1] Since that time survival rates of 80 percent have been reported in various microsurgical centers around the world.[2-6] The improved survival rate reflects the increased sophistication of microsurgical instruments and techniques, the experience amassed by many microsurgeons, and the development of well coordinated microsurgical teams working in specialized centers. The simultaneous advancement in free tissue transplantation has expanded the scope of possibilities open to the microsurgeon in replantation of the upper extremity.

Emerging from this decade of surgical-technological development is the recognition that the full potential, with regard to rehabilitation and functional restoration of replanted limbs, has yet to be explored. Progress along functional lines has already been made on a broad front and is largely attributable to refined standards of indications and contraindications based on cumulative past experience. Equally important is the recognition of a coordinated team approach between surgeons and skilled hand therapists. The hand therapist must be well versed in the overall concepts of hand surgery, wound healing, and treatment, as well as possessing a working knowledge of the unique problems that are encountered with a replantation patient.

A review of the surgical considerations[2-5,7-9] and techniques as well as principles of wound healing[7,10-13] is essential in understanding the unique problems that are presented to the therapist when treating a limb that has been replanted.

SURGICAL CONSIDERATIONS

The sophistication of microsurgical techniques and the development of instrumentation has led to the increasing success of reattachment surgery. Indications and contraindications for replantation[2,5,7,9,11,14] are now more clearly defined, although they are not absolute. The decision to replant is relative to many factors.

91

A.   The general condition of the patient must be considered in order to determine whether there is an acceptable risk of undergoing a long and complex surgical procedure. Pre-existing general health problems such as heart disease or diabetes may preclude replantation. Any concomitant life-threatening injury takes priority.

B.   The type of injury is closely related to the prognosis for survival and ultimate function. Survival is most dependent upon the vascular repairs, whereas function relates more closely to nerve regeneration and favorable scar formation. Both are influenced by the type of injury. A detailed history of how the accident occurred is important in determining the full extent of injury. The type of device that caused the injury, the forces involved, the contact surface, and space in which the part was caught, as well as exposure to temperature extremes will help to determine the extent of tissue damage.

C.   The condition of the amputated part should be such that reasonably good functional recovery can be predicted, rather than survival alone.

Common types of injuries are guillotine, local crush, severe crush, or avulsion. The guillotine-type injury is produced by sharp objects. Tissue damage is minimal and limited to the cut ends. As long as the ischemic period is not prolonged, the prognosis is good, particularly at distal levels where nerve regeneration is more favorable. Local crush or compression injuries also tend toward a favorable prognosis, as tissue damage is limited to a short distance proximal and distal to the amputation. An example is a punch press injury. This type of injury necessitates more extensive debridement and bone shortening, thus making functional recovery less favorable than for a guillotine-type injury.

A severe diffuse crush or an avulsion injury results in extensive tissue damage, much of which is not readily apparent. Such injuries are the result of a blunt trauma, often accompanied by rotational forces that tear rather than cut the tissue. Multiple level injury can result, with extensive internal damage. There is a high frequency of thrombosis and tissue necrosis, even if circulation can be established initially. Survival and return of useful function is questionable.

D.   Duration of anoxia. Prompt and effective cooling of the amputated part will minimize irreversible cellular damage. The ideal temperature for tissue preservation is 2 to 4°C.[7] Large muscle masses are most susceptible to tissue necrosis; irreversible damage occurs after 6 hours of warm ischemic time.[5,7,9] Parts with little or no muscle tissue tolerate anoxia for longer periods (8 to 10 hours).[7] Digits have been reported to survive for 20 hours following proper cooling techniques.[5,7] Effective cooling of digits is best accomplished by placing the parts in a plastic bag to keep them dry and then immersing the the bag in a container of water and ice. The parts must not be frozen, or tissue damage will result, similiar to a frostbite injury. Packing the digits on ice alone will freeze the tissue.

E.   Level of amputation. High-level amputations are associated with life-threatening problems due to profuse blood loss, the larger muscle masses involved, the possibility of toxic metabolic complications, and the frequency of occurrence of other injury. From a technical standpoint, the surgery itself may pose fewer difficulties, however; functionally the arm is dependent upon nerve regeneration which has a poorer prognosis with higher level injuries. With digital amputations, greater labor, time, and skill are needed due to the small and complex structures the surgeon must repair. The potential for nerve regeneration is often greater, due to the shorter distances involved. Multiple levels of injury are generally not considered for replantation unless the thumb is involved, in which case every attempt is made to save usable parts. Even if metacarpophalangeal and interphalangeal motion are lost, the thumb can function well with some degree of carpometacarpal mobility.

From a functional standpoint, the lower forearm and wrist amputation is a prime candidate for reattachment. At this level muscle mass is minimal, the flexors and extensors are tendinous, and excellent nerve regeneration can be expected due to the relatively short distance that is required to reinnervate the hand intrinsics and sensory end organs.

Humeral amputations pose life-threatening problems, as well as a much poorer prognosis for nerve regneration and recovery of useful function. Upper forearm amputation is frequently associated with extensive muscle loss of the flexors and extensors. Amputations across the metacarpals often necessitate secondary procedures such as tenolysis and capsulotomies, but still tend toward favorable functional restoration. Digital amputations require much individualized consideration, as many factors influence the decision whether or not to replant. In order to be used for gripping objects securely, the fingers require a good flexion arc, particularly of digits three, four, and five. The second digit is used mainly for finer prehensile activities, and thus a decreased flexion arc is not as great a hindrance to good function, particularly when metacarpophalangeal motion is good. Amputations proximal to the insertion of the flexor digitorum superficialis will usually result in greater restriction of the flexion arc, and thus will lead to a poorer functional result. Amputations distal to its insertion result in decreased DIP motion, which is functionally less significant than PIP flexion. With amputations in close proximity to the PIP joint, arthrodesis of the joint in a functional flexed position should be considered as useful; painfree joint motion is rarely obtained. If a single digit has a poor chance of sensory recovery, coupled with extensive damage of the joints, reattachment should not be attempted, as these digits end up only getting in the way, limiting overall hand function, and increasing the risk of future injury. Many patients favor all attempts toward reattachment, despite prognosis for poor function, due to the value they place on the cosmetic result. From the authors' experience, patients have regained good function from a badly mutilated hand but refuse to use it in public due to its appearance. These realities must be kept in mind when the surgeon decides whether or not to replant a part and/or attempt salvage replantation surgery.

TECHNIQUE OF REPLANTATION

Technical information is beyond the scope of this chapter; however, an overview will be presented to familiarize the therapist with the general procedure of replantation.

Once the patient has been admitted to the replantation center, work is immediately begun on the amputated parts. X-rays are taken to determine whether lower bony injury is present. One team of surgeons begin locating and tagging all structures to permit rapid identification during repair. General anesthesia is most often used, and tourniquets are placed around the upper arm and opposite lower limb, in case vein grafts are needed. Meticulous debridement of all devitalized tissue is critical to prevent thrombosis, infection, and excessive scarring, which contributes to greater immobility. Vessels, skin, and soft tissues are cut back to healthy areas. One team of surgeons prepares the stump while the other prepares the amputated part.

Bone shortening is often necessary to eliminate undue tension on the neurovascular repairs. Nerve grafts are utilized to repair large gaps. If bone shortening is required, care must be taken to match the length of the tendons, nerves, and vessels to insure proper excursion during active movement. Rigid internal fixation is critical in achieving stabilization of the extremity so that early motion of adjacent joints can be initiated in therapy. Inadequate fixation leads to movement in the vascular unions and angulation or rotation of the part. A combination of Kirschner wires, screws, circumflage wires, or intermedullar plates is used to acheive fixation.

Following bony fixation, the order of repairs depends upon the level of amputation, deeper structures being repaired first. The exception is when blood loss has been extensive; then efforts are made to restore circulation first. Survival of the part depends upon exacting repair of the vascular structures. Accurate nerve repair will greatly determine how the limb will function. If a clear division of the nerve is present without retraction and the nerve ends can be approximated, then a primary repair is carried out. If extensive gaps in the nerve are present, then nerve grafts are utilized. The goal of tendon repair is complete union whenever possible, so that early mobilization can be initiated to prevent stiff joints. If extensive tendon damage is present, then secondary repair with insertion of silicone rods for two-stage tendon grafting is done. The flexor tendons take priority over the extensor tendons because of their importance in functional grip patterns. Also, they can tolerate tension earlier than the extensors, thus allowing earlier active motion, which, in turn, helps to prevent joint stiffness.

Skin closure is the last step in the surgical process. If the skin can be approximated without excessive tension, then it is sutured, taking care to suture loosely over the dorsum of the hand to prevent vascular constriction produced by edema. With forearm replantation, a fasciotomy of the forearm is done to release pressure caused by edema within the muscle compartments, which would lead to vascular constriction and subsequent muscle necrosis similar to a Volkmann's ischemia. At the wrist level, a carpal tunnel release is necessary to avoid compression to the median nerve secondary to edema. At both of these levels, it is common to close the wounds using a single thickness skin graft for temporary closure. This allows additional room for the edema, which can be profuse, and prevents added constriction on the vessels. Once edema has decreased and rehabilitation has progressed to the point where the joints regain mobility, this graft can be removed for more cosmetic closure. Pedicle grafts or free flaps are used when skin loss is great or when a good cover of soft tissue is needed over tendon repairs. Frequently single thickness or mesh grafts are used, primarily to close the wound, particularly if there is a question about potential viability of the vascular anastomosis and greater risk of infection or other complications which might necessitate reexploration. They are later replaced with pedicle or free flap grafts.

Skin over the dorsum of the hand is loose and can be manually pulled away from underlying structures. This allows greater mobility of metacarpophalangeal (MCP) range of motion, as grafts tend to be less elastic than the original skin and often bind down to the superficial extensor tendons. Free flaps or pedicle grafts over this area allow unrestricted MCP range of motion and are therefore better suited.

EARLY POST-OPERATIVE MANAGEMENT

Postoperatively, antibacterial ointments are used over the wound, and bulky supportive non-adherent compressive dressings are applied. The hand is supported by a cast, with the tips free to enable close monitoring of any color changes indicative of thrombosis. Manipulation is kept at a minimum. The dressings are left in place, untouched for at least 1 week post-replantation, in the digits. At more proximal levels, the dressings may be lighter and may be changed more frequently to allow early detection of necrosis or infection.

Elevation and immobilization are mandatory immediately postoperatively. The period of immobilization varies from patient to patient. Good internal fixation is necessary in order to allow early mobilization in the rehabilitation program. Traditionally, 2 to 3 weeks of immobilization were recommended for a digit and 4 to 6 weeks for the limb. Recently, earlier mobilization has been advocated in a very controlled fashion, supervised by an experienced hand therapist. The risk of tendon rupture must be accepted if this approach is adopted. Given the number of structures damaged in close proximity, the resultant swelling and collagen proliferation, the authors have found that the longer the period of immobilization, the greater the resultant range of motion deficits and subsequent functional deficit. Therefore, fewer problems with joint stiffness result when therapy is begun early, i.e., the second postoperative week for a digit and the third or fourth week for a more proximal wound.

WOUND HEALING

Knowledge of wound healing is critical to understanding the rationale behind the therapy regime utilized with the replant patient, and must therefore precede any discussion of rehabilitative management. For specific information on the wound healing process and the stages of wound healing and scar maturation, the authors direct you to chapter 1.

Therapy protocols have been published for soft tissue, tendon,[15,16] nerve,[7] and bony injuries[17]; however, little information to date has been published on the management of the unique and complex problems encountered when treating the replantation patient. Functional restoration of these patients can be very challenging when every structure has been damaged (bone, tendon, nerve, vessels, and soft tissue). Each tissue requires a different period of immobilization; therefore it is essential that the evaluation and therapy regime be based on the healing times of the various tissues involved.

Care must be taken to apply the appropriate degree of stress at the optimal stage of healing to avoid rupture or microtears around the repaired structure, which in turn leads to increased scar and adhesion formation. Guidelines for wound healing of each structure are documented[12,13]; however, it must be emphasized that there are no cookbook answers to indicate when to begin to stress each tissue. A coordinated effort in the decision making process between surgeon and hand therapist is most effective. The surgeon is the most familiar with each individual patient's surgical status and, therefore, during the initial stages of wound healing, must ultimately decide when therapy can be initiated and at what point each structure can be stressed.

The skin is usually the first tissue that can be mobilized. Sutured skin has adequate tensile strength after 7 to 10 days to allow the removal of stitches.[17] Grafted skin may need special care and additional healing time to ensure viable circulation.

The vascular supply requires 14 days to heal.[17] During this time, elevation of the extremity is important to minimize edema, which can cause excess pressure on the vascular repairs. A bulky, supportive dressing is left in place, uninterrupted for 7 days. Care must be taken to avoid constriction of the vessels by bandaging and casting too tightly.

The nerves are healed at 3 to 4 weeks.[7] Two important factors that affect the success of the nerve repair are excessive stretch and compression on the nerve. Excessive stretch increases the scar formation, which may block axonal regeneration. It is critical to achieve a nerve repair without tension. Regeneration occurs more effectively through two suture lines produced by nerve grafting versus one suture line under tension. Postoperatively, the repair should be protected by casting the part in a relaxed position, but not in excessive flexion, which can result in a stretch injury once mobilization begins.[7] Compression should be avoided when bandaging, casting, and subsequent splinting, as it can also delay axonal regeneration.

The classic causes for delay of fracture healing with or without the formation of a pseudoarthrosis are largely related to medical and environmental factors, most of which are outside the realm of the hand therapist's control. Failure to obtain complete reduction and adequate fixation results in the interposition of soft tissue between the bone ends, resulting in the development of a non-union. Loss of bony substance after a severe wound such as a gun shot wound results in loss of stability at the fracture site.

When discussing successful wound healing, one must view it in terms of the final outcome, which is, hopefully, a well-functioning extremity. The replant patient is at a definite disadvantage, due to the number of structures that must undergo repair in such close proximity. Active collagen synthesis is taking place concomitantly in the bone, tendons, nerve, vessels, and skin. Edema can be profuse, whereas a more localized edema is associated with less severe trauma.

Individual structures have a tendency to adhere to whatever structures are adjacent. For example, it is common for the flexor tendons to adhere to the bone in a replantation of the proximal phalanx. Prolonged immobilization to ensure good bone healing will jeopardize the mobility of the joints and tendon gliding, resulting in a stiff, immobile hand.

Surgical and therapy protocols for the replantation patient must not be solely based on the repair and healing of isolated structes, but on the regeneration that is taking place throughout the replanted part. This total healing process will influence the functional outcome.

EARLY THERAPY PHASE

Before therapy can be initiated, the therapist must be familiar with the patient's history and surgical report. It is important to know the date of surgery, type of injury (crush, avulsion, or guillotine), level of injury of each structure, bony fixation, and wound closure procedures utilized.

The early therapy phase, from 0 to 4 weeks, is oriented toward protecting repairs, wound healing, edema control, and early mobilization. The cast is removed and x-rays are taken to evaluate the extent of bony healing and to determine whether the pins can be removed. Then the therapist fabricates a positioning splint to protect the bony unions and tendon repairs. The wrist is positioned in neutral to avoid undue stress on the flexor and extensor repairs. The MCP joints and PIP joints are often difficult to position due to edema, pain, and joint stiffness. The MCP joints should be positioned in flexion and the IP joints in only slight flexion to maintain the length of the collateral ligaments at these joints.

At this time, the patient is issued written instructions on the care, wearing time, and precautions with the splint, as well as written instruction in a wound care program. We find that written instructions to reinforce what was verbalized help a great deal in follow-through at home. Frequently, this initial visit can be very traumatic for the patient. It is the first time that the bandages have been removed since the initial surgery. The patient may have a preconceived notion that the hand will look and function as it did prior to the accident. A certain amount of discomfort is experienced during cast and bandage removal. If pins are removed, many patients feel the fingers will fall off during this process. As a result of the emotional and physical trauma the person is experiencing, the person may not fully absorb the verbal instructions given to them. It is important for the therapist to keep instructions simple, to inform a responsible family member as well as the patient, and to offer reassurance and support to both the patient and family members.

Ideally, the next therapy visit should be 1 or 2 days following fabrication of the protective splint, so that the splint can be checked and adjusted if necessary, and to determine how well the patient is able to carry through with the wound care program.

WOUND MANAGEMENT

The first problem to be dealt with is wound healing. The patient may have sutures, K-wires, or pins in place. Depending on the type of injury, the skin may be open in areas, sutured, or grafted. An important goal of wound healing is to avoid infection. The wound care program will vary, depending upon the type of wound closure. If the wound is sutured closed and pins are in place, soaking the hand is avoided. Sutures and pins are internal routes for infection. The whirlpool can be used for a few sessions, just to clean the hand after the cast is removed; however, prolonged use may increase edema and the risk of infection. It is recommended that the patient wash the hand two to three times per day with soap and water rather than soaking, pat it dry, and apply peroxide or betadine around the pin and sutures. The hand should then be bandaged with a clean dry gauze. Pin track infections can necessitate removal of the pins before healing is adequate, thus increasing the chance of nonunion or malunion of the fracture site.

If open wounds are present, whirlpool treatments become necessary to cleanse the wound and loosen necrotic tissue prior to debridement. Betadine is added to the water, and treatments do not exceed 20 minutes, as prolonged positioning in the dependent position will increase edema.[18,19] The patient is encouraged to actively move his hand to counteract the effects of edema. Careful debridement of necrotic tissue follows each whirlpool session. The wound is then either dressed with a dry sterile gauze or coated with Silvadene or an alternate antibacterial cream, depending on the instructions from the surgeon.

The whirlpool should be avoided with grafted skin, as the skin can become macerated, thus interferring with the viability of the graft. Once viability is assured, a few sessions of whirlpool to loosen necrotic tissue may be necessary. Xeroform* is commonly used to dress the grafted area so as not to disrupt the graft when redressing the wound.

Home wound care instruction is critical to avoid infection. Infections can cause increased scarring and adhesion formation around repaired structures. Depending on the severity, immediate hospitalization with IV antibiotics may be necessary, which, in turn, delays the beginning of therapy sessions. Much valuable time may be lost in combatting infection.

THE VALUE OF MOBILIZATION

Once the cast has been removed, a protective splint fabricated, and wound care addressed, a more dynamic approach can be initiated, usually 2 to 5 weeks after replantation. At this stage, it is important to begin moving all joints that are not fixated.

The effect of immobilization on joints has been well documented. Evans and Edgar[20] studied the effects of immobilization and remobilization of rat knee joints and identified the following causes of joint stiffness after immobilization: contracture of muscle and joint capsule, proliferation of intracapusular connective tissue and adhesion formation, and major cartilage alterations. Immobilization also interferes with cartilage nutrition. Synovial fluid is a main source of cartilage nutrition, and diffusion of this fluid through articular cartilage is aided by intermittent compression of the cartilage during movement.[21]

The effects of immobilization cited above were studied on nontraumatized joints. These effects are substantially exacerbated in the traumatized joints and tissues that are found with replantation. Peacock[9] cites the fact that an immobilized joint that is surrounded by edematous soft tissue will become stiff faster and more severely. Cartilage damage can be expected when K-wires are passed through joints for bony fixation or if there are interarticular fractures. Ruback[21] has found that articular cartilage defects heal with connective tissue rather than through the synthesis of hyaline cartilage, when immobilized for only 3 weeks.

Although the replantation patient may be started on therapy within the first 2 to 3 weeks post-surgery, the repaired structures have not developed enough tensile strength to tolerate active movement. The techniques of joint mobilization are of great value at this point. Grade I and II accessory and physiological movements can aid to preserve gliding of joint surfaces without putting tension on the tendon or neurovascular structures, which may not be ready to be mobilized.

The effects of early motion have been documented. Salter[22] observed that defects

---

*Xeroform, Cheeseborough-Ponds, Inc, Hospital Products Division, Greenwich, CT 06830

in articular cartilage were filled with hyaline cartilage rather than fibrous tissue when the joint surfaces were passively moved during the healing process. Akeson[23] found that motion prevents the haystack orientation of new collagen fibers which inhibits movement. Mobilization has also been found to decrease chondrofibrosis, which can ankylose joints in interarticular fractures.[13]

Attention should be given to proximal joints. Frequently, due to anxiety about getting knocked, the patient will hold the extremity close to the body in the position of protection, i.e., shoulder internally rotated and adducted, elbow flexed, wrist flexed with MCP's extended, IPs flexed, and thumb adducted. This position is opposite the position of function and can result in shoulder and elbow stiffness and pain, as well as tightening of the MCP and IP collateral ligaments. The protective splint will serve to counteract this posture in the hand. The patient must be instructed to AROM exercises for all uninvolved proximal joints to prevent a frozen shoulder, elbow flexion contracture, and stiffness of the non-fixated joints.

EARLY ADL INTERVENTION

Attention must also be given to early ADL evaluation and training, particularly if the patient lives alone. With the hand splinted in a protective position, encourage the patient to use it as a gross stabilizer to assist the uninvolved hand. Adaptive equipment may be appropriate to encourage independence initially; however, as the period of immobilization ends, encourage the patient to begin using his replanted part for as many simple, non-stressful activities as possible. In the beginning, activity may be restricted to supervised activities in the clinic and progress to tasks at home. Early activity orientation helps the patient to overcome the fear that the hand will fall off, as well as encouraging gentle active joint movement. This approach helps the patient to reintegrate the injured part back into his body image versus viewing it as a separate entity from the rest of his body.

The patient's splinting needs are evaluated. The protective splint is adjusted to accommodate increasing ROM, with emphasis on MCP flexion and PIP extension. The patient now wears the splint overnight to maintain good positioning and in situations where he is at high risk for getting knocked or bumped into during the day. Dynamic splinting to encourage gentle active ROM is begun. Traction splinting to increase passive joint movement is still contraindicated. The actual splint design will depend upon the level of injury. An outrigger extension assist splint is fabricated for a hand replantation of the lower forearm, wrist, or palmar level. The purpose of the splint is to promote tendon gliding and early joint movement. The rationale for its use is that the flexor tendons heal before the extensor tendons and can tolerate tension earlier. The splint gives a gentle opposing force to the flexors during the range, while assisting the extensors. The extensors remain relaxed, based upon the principle of reciprocal inhibition. Therefore, tendon gliding is achieved without stressing the extensors. Joint movement is both guided and encouraged, to prevent adhesions. Nutrition and blood supply to the tendons are enhanced. The authors have not observed extensor tendon rupture with this technique. The surgeons feel that the risk of rupture is less critical than the risk of stiff joints.

The splint is volar based to achieve greater support of the hand and its arches and to provide a base for traction outriggers to increase joint flexion once passive ROM can be initiated. If clawing due to loss of lumbrical function results, then a dorsal based splint with a lumbrical stop can serve as the base for the extension assist outrigger.

For digital replantations, joint movement should be assessed in order to determine whether the splint will be based on the hand or the digit. If MCP motion is normal, then this joint can be blocked in neutral to allow active ROM (AROM) forces to be transferred to the PIP and DIP joints.

Care must be taken not to compromise circulation in the replanted part. Splints should be designed to increase the surface area of contact with the skin in order to distribute pressure evenly and to avoid constriction of the venous return and further edema. Early edema control is important, as mentioned in other chapters. The methods that seem most effective are elevation, external force or compression, and the internal force or compression of muscular contraction produced by active exercise.[11,18] Measurements are taken in order to accurately assess the effectiveness of treatment techniques used to decrease edema. Initially, the patient is instructed to elevate the part as much as possible. The DePuy elevation pillow* has been used effectively overnight, as has an elevation sling attached to an IV pole or suspended from a screw-eye attached into the ceiling.

Massage techniques are taught to the patient. As much AROM as is allowed at each stage is encouraged, as well as the use of the exercise splint to restore the pumping action to the muscles. Once the wound is healed, edema reduction techniques become more aggressive with the use of Isotoner gloves,** Jobst garments, and Coban† wrappings. The Jobst (intermittent compression) unit with its distal to proximal pressure gradient has also been effective, particularly with arm and hand replants. Cord wrapping can be used to produce a quick but temporary decrease in edema prior to AROM exercises, in order to maximize gains made within a therapy session.

Use of the Jobst jet air splint‡ (a more portable version of the compression unit) enables the patient to carry through at home with the program of edema reduction. The clear plastic allows close monitoring of color changes in the hand and can be easily adjusted by the patient to avoid venous constriction.

LATE PHASE EVALUATION AND TREATMENT (5 TO 8 WEEKS)

Late phase of treatment for the replanted part is aimed at stressing the hand to maximize joint mobility, tendon excursion, and overall functional use of the hand. It is generally begun in a graded fashion at 6 to 8 weeks post-replantation, once the fractures are stable and tendons and neurovascular structures are healed. A thorough hand evaluation preceeds this stage of treatment, in order to establish a baseline of perfor-

---

*DePuy Prokop Co, P.O. Box 816, Rockville Center, NY 11570.
**Jobst Co, Box 653, Toledo, OH 43694.
†Coban, 3M Corp, Medical Products Division, St Paul, MN 55101.
‡Jobst Co, Box 653, Toledo, OH 43694.

mance. Passive and active ROM at each joint is evaluated, using goniometric measurements. A total AROM measurement is also taken by having the patient approximate a fist and measuring the number of centimeters between the tip of the distal phalanx and the distal palmar crease. The digit-o-meter* (a plastic measuring device calibrated in centimeters) can be used for ease in measuring. This method is a quick, easy way to assess the functional AROM available in each digit, and can be communicated quite easily to the surgeons when they inquire about the progress the patient is making.

A manual muscle test is now appropriate, as are functional prehension strength measurements obtained with the dynamometer and pinch meter. We find that strength measurements obtained for gross grasp, palmar, lateral and tip pinch are much better indicators of potential functional strength in the hand than is the traditional manual muscle test. Frequently a patient may obtain satisfactory grades when testing individual muscles, but score quite low on tests of grip strength and have difficulty performing many prehension activities. Factors that affect this outcome are inherent in the manual muscle test itself. Muscles in the forearm and hand work in synergy to produce gripping power, not in an isolated fashion. For example, when testing a given muscle, adjacent joints may be stabilized in recommended positions, i.e., when testing the long finger flexors, the wrist is held in neutral. This stabilization is lacking when squeezing the dynamometer. If there is pain, weakness, or instability at the wrist, the reading on the dynamometer may read zero, despite the fact that the sublimus and profundus muscles response for finger flexion test good or good plus.

This phenomenon is common with wrist fractures and radial nerve palsies. Another factor that commonly pertains to the replant patient is that the strength may be good, but in a very limited range due to joint tightness or tendon adhesions, thus producing ineffective grasp when prehending either a dynamometer or an object. In essence, the functional prehension strength measures give a more accurate assessment of what the patient's hand function will be like; the manual muscle test is useful in assessing when particular muscles are being reinnervated. Changes in strength should be documented to monitor nerve regeneration and muscle reinnervation. In addition to actual strength measurements, the patient will be asked to perform a number of activities that require gross grasp, palmar, lateral, and tip pinch. They are graded on whether or not they can prehend the object in the typical manner or whether substitutions are utilized. A few representative activities include holding a hammer, throwing a ball, picking up a pencil and coins, and turning a key in a lock. All evaluations are repeated on a monthly basis in order to keep accurate records of the patient's progress. Once progress has plateaued for a number of consecutive evaluations, the surgeon may then consider additional surgical procedures, such as capsulotomies or tenolysis.

During this phase of treatment, therapy becomes more directed. The main emphasis is to influence scar formation, as unfavorable scar interferes with all phases of restorative hand surgery, whether it be tendon gliding, joint motion, nerve regeneration, or skin compliance. At this stage of treatment, collagen synthesis has taken place. But now the scar requires the appropriate stress to realign the fibers in a longitudinal manner, versus the initial haphazard arrangement. Unfavorable scar adhesions interfere with tendon gliding. Repaired tendons may fail to glide because the adhesions undergo

---

*Fred Sammons, Inc., Box 32, Brookfield, IL 60513-0032

remodeling that produces an unfavorable, non-yielding, dense scar. Postoperative rehabilitation techniques are based on stressing the scar to influence the remodelling process to produce a more favorable filmy, loose adhesion between the tendon and its surrounding structures that will permit tendon gliding. Scar can also limit joint motion by interfering with the intracapsular and extracapsular movements associated with normal joint function. Nerve regeneration is limited by scar formation between the nerve ends, thus inhibiting motor and sensory function in the hand. Scar in skin can produce severe contractures across flexion creases, which interfere with tendon gliding and joint motion.

All grades of joint mobilization are now tolerated, as well as passive stretching in the form of manual stretch and static and dynamic traction splinting. Splint designs for replanted parts may be complex due to the multiplicity of structures damaged and the levels of injury. The patient may need splinting to increase passive and active ROM in flexion and extension at various joints. Frequently the thumb must be included. As a result, one splint is made to perform many functions. A typical splint for a hand replant patient may be a volar splint with MP and PIP traction into flexion and dorsal outrigger to encourage AROM, into flexion (Fig. 5-1). In addition, for the thumb, both volar and dorsal outriggers may be added to increase passive flexion and to encourage AROM into flexion, respectively. The patient may need traction splinting to increase passive extension as well, which would involve a dorsal-based traction splint.

Splints for flexion and extension are alternated throughout the day with exercise between splinting sessions. The patient will also wear a static splint overnight to main-

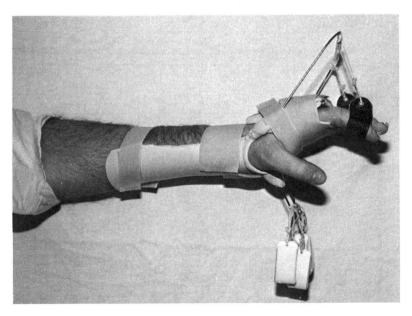

Fig. 5-1.   This patient is status post-replantation of digits 2–4, with partial amputation of digit 5. The dorsal outrigger is used to encourage active ROM of each digit at the proximal interphalangeal joint. This acts to preserve gliding of both flexor and extensor tendons.

tain ROM gains made during the day. The splint may position the digits in either flexion or extension, depending upon which deficit appears to interfere with function the most.

Frequently, with digital replantations distal to the MCP joint, the joint may regain normal ROM fairly quickly. In order to increase flexion at the IP joints, the MP joints may need to be blocked in extension so the flexion forces will be transmitted to the IP joints (Fig. 5-2).

The authors have found that elastomer* inserts worn underneath the splint but molded over an area of dense scar are very effective in softening scar tissue so that it can be stretched more easily. Splints will vary widely, depending upon the level of injury and the joints affected. Our splinting approach is based on a problem-oriented method, i.e., we assess limitations at each joint as well as how more proximal joint positions affect distal contractures. We also assess if a ROM limitation is due to joint tightness, tendon adhesion, or skin contracture and splint accordingly.

Our philosophy of splinting any injured hand, particularly the replanted hand is to look at each individual's splinting needs as unique. We do not select a splint for a patient based on a preconceived idea about which splint is appropriate for that diagnosis, but thoroughly evaluate the specific factors that limit the patient's ability to move his hand in a functional manner. This philosophy precludes many prefabricated hand splints. Hands do not come in small-medium-large. Many patients who have had re-

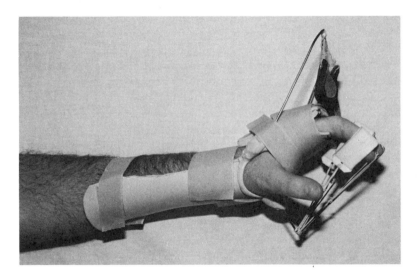

Fig. 5-2. Once the extensors can tolerate stretching into flexion, a volar outrigger is added to increase flexion at the interphalangeal joints. Metacarpal phalangeal joint range of motion is within normal limits, therefore the splint blocks the MCPs in extension, allowing the full traction force to be transmitted to the interphalangeal joints, which lack range. The patient can actively extend against the force of the rubberbands once the extensors can withstand resistance.

---

*WFR Corp, PO Box 215, Ramsey, NJ 07446

plantations may have large free flap or pedicle grafts, which necessitate custom fits. Since only the main blood vessels are sutured, much of the collateral circulation to a part remains interrupted and needs sufficient time to become re-established. As a result, care must be taken to achieve a good, comfortable fit without vascular constriction. It is difficult to do this with prefabricated splints. Some prefabricated splints are useful for digital replantations. The LMB wirefoam PIP extension splints* and Capener† splints work well to increase passive extension, while allowing resisted flexion. The leather PIP and DIP flexion straps help to improve flexion, but are only useful for the end degrees of range. Buddy straps are frequently used to attach a digit with poor ROM to one that has good AROM, in order to help increase the PROM of the digit that lacks range.

For more severe contractures at the PIP joint, hand-based outrigger traction may be required to increase passive ROM. Written instructions accompany all splints, and patients are encouraged to bring splints to each therapy session, as frequent adjustments are necessary as improvements are note.

Graded resistive prehension activities, as well as manipulative tasks, are also begun at this time in order to stress the hand. We find the beginning of this phase to be a critical time that influences the ultimate function the hand will obtain. The patient is taught how to use whatever motion is available to assist himself with activities of daily living. Repeated hand function and ADL evaluations will help to pinpoint specific deficit areas that should be addressed. Activities are chosen to simulate work-related tasks. Activities that involve tool manipulation and use, such as woodworking, plumbing, and electrical projects are emphasized for tradesmen. Kitchen, gardening, and craft activities are utilized when appropriate.

For stress to be most effective, it should be applied before significant adhesions form about each structure. After weeks of immobilization or minimal activity, the scar will undoubtedly heal unfavorably. Two or three sessions of therapy a week cannot provide sufficient stress to influence the remodeling process adequately. The patient must take responsibility for working the hand intermittently throughout the day, every day. Particularly at this stage, if the patient makes minimal effort to move the hand or if stress is inadequate, there will be little gain in tendon gliding and joint movement. The therapist's role is to guide the patient in appropriate exercises and activities to be carried out at home. ROM and functional gains achieved in therapy will be temporary at best, unless the patient assumes an active role in his rehabilitation. Therapy putty, grippers, and weights are used as an adjunct to hands-on therapy and provide an excellent means for the patient to stress his hand at home.

The functional significance of cutaneous sensibility of the hand is well recognized. The dexterity, coordination, and skill of the human hand is dependent on normal sensory function. Even if muscle power is adequate, the hand may not be used if sensation is lacking. In general, it has been our experience that those who have functional sensation are more likely to return to work and view their replantations more positively. If the patient has to constantly visually monitor their hand during activities, due to poor sensation, they are less likely to use it spontaneously. As sensation is such an

---

*LMB Hand Rehab Products, 111 Nieto Ave., Long Beach, CA 90803.
†Roylan Manufacturing Co, Inc, PO Box 555, Menomonee Falls, WI 53051.

important part of the overall hand function, and we are interested particularly in the extent to which the replantation patient achieves sensory recovery, we do a comprehensive sensory evaluation. Our aim is to establish a baseline of the quality of sensation present in the hand, i.e., anesthetic, protective, or epicritic, and to chart the progression of sensory recovery. Information obtained is used to educate the patient as to deficit areas and precautionary measures to avoid injury, to assist the surgeon in determining whether neurolysis would be of benefit, and to determine at what point the patient would benefit from a program of sensory re-education.

The tests we administer are designed to give us information on constant touch, which is mediated by the slowly adapting fiber receptor system, and moving touch, mediated by the quickly adapting fiber receptor system. (See Ch. 3 for additional information on sensory measurement.) Initial testing is delayed until wounds are healed, edema is reduced, and the patient's hand is free of scaly skin. This delay usually corresponds to the lag time that occurs in the growth of axons following a nerve injury, approximately one month post-replantation. We administer the tests in an order based on the sensory reinnervation pattern documented by Dellon.[10] After noting the scars, Tinel's sign, and pseudomotor function, we have the patient do a sensory mapping of the hand to give us an idea of where to start our testing. We procede with tests of hotcold, 30 c/s vibration, moving touch, deep touch, 256 cps of vibration, moving two-point discrimination, and static two-point discrimination. Testing is done bimonthly.

As sensation returns, the patient experiences paresthesias with complaints of tingling, electric shock sensations, and cold intolerance. This hypersensitivity syndrome is dealt with using graded sensory bombardment to encourage adaptation to the sensory input as the nerve matures.

A variety of textured materials are used to stimulate the area, such as fabrics (toweling, velvet, burlap); food textures (rice, lentils, macaroni, kidney beans); and object manipulation to build up tolerance to pressure. Tapping, brushing, massaging, and eventually vibration can be tolerated. The patient applies all stimuli to himself and is encouraged to work for 10-minute periods four to five times per day. With this graded program initiated early in the treatment, we have avoided long-term hypersensitivity problems. Once hypersensitivity has decreased and sensory testing reveals 30 c/s of vibration and moving touch to be intact, we begin a concentrated sensory re-education program.

"Sensory re-education cannot induce axonal regeneration, but it has been well documented that sensory re-education can help the patient achieve the fullest potential provided by the nerve repair."[10] The method involves implementation of specific sensory exercises at the appropriate stages of nerve regeneration. Please refer to the section on sensory re-education found in Chapter 3 for specific re-education techniques.

VOCATIONAL PSYCHO-SOCIAL ASPECT OF REPLANTATION

The majority of our patients are injured on the job and may not be able to return to the same job. Some patients may have to accept lighter duty with the same company, or change jobs, which would require an alteration in the work environment. This, of course, depends upon whether or not the company is willing to make needed changes to accommodate their employee.

We refer all patients to the vocational counseling department early in the rehabilitative process. Job alternatives are discussed, and we try to focus the patient on returning to some form of work as soon as possible. Restorative activites are designed to simulate work tasks. The vocational counselor then makes contact with the employer to assess the responsiveness of the employer to the employee's needs. On occasion, the therapist will perform a site visit with the vocational counselor, employer, and patient to see whether the patient has the hand function required to perform the job and to make suggestions on possible alternatives to performing particular aspects of the job. We find that those who do return to work soon after injury, even if the job has been modified to some degree to eliminate heavy resistive tasks, tend ultimately to adjust better to their disability.

Psychologically, each patient seems to handle their disability differently. Some are motivated to work hard and return to work as soon as possible. Others are content to extend their period of unemployment. A certain percentage attend therapy with a preconceived idea that they will receive large settlements as a result of their injury, and therefore they refuse vocational counseling. Large settlements rarely occur, and the patient is the one who ultimately is the loser.

Some patients view cosmesis as being more important than function. We have had patients with badly mutilated hands who can do many activities with the hand and do so in public. Others with relatively minor injuries may keep the hand in their pocket and use it only in private, if at all. Despite the varied results obtained with these patients and the sometimes lengthy rehabilitation, all but one of our patients ultimately chose amputation rather than replantation.

CASE STUDY 1

The patient is a 31-year-old female, status post left upper extremity replantation at the mid-humeral level (Fig. 5-3). Amputation occurred when a driver lost control of his car and collided with a stop sign that sheared off the patient's arm in a guillotine fashion. X-ray revealed a fractured ulna, which occurred when the amputated extremity fell to the ground. Both fractures were fixated with rods. All structures were repaired. The median nerve had retracted into the axilla, thus requiring nerve grafting for primary repair. Ischemic time was 4 to 5 hours. A forearm fasciotomy and carpal tunnel release were performed, and skin grafts were used to cover the forearm wound (Fig. 5-4). The patient was discharged from the hospital 5 weeks post-replantation.

The early phase rehabilitation was based on a problem-oriented approach, many areas being addressed simultaneously (Fig. 5-5). She had severe pitting edema. Her arm was wrapped in an ace bandage, and an isotoner glove was fitted to her hand. A Jobst compression unit was used daily prior to each treatment. Her arm was elevated on pillows overnight, and she used a sling during the day. She was issued a Jobst full arm jet air splint to be used at home intermittently to maintain the gains made by the compression unit used in the clinic. As swelling de-

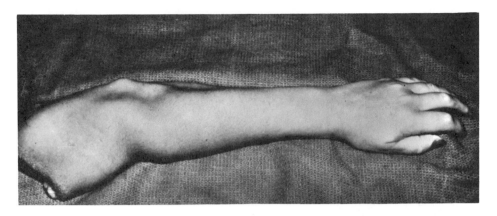

Fig. 5-3. Dorsal view. Amputation occurred in a guillotine fashion at the mid-humeral level of the left dominant upper extremity. (Slide compliments of William Shaw, MD, and Stephen Colen, MD.)

creased and wounds were healed, she was fitted with a Jobst arm sleeve and glove.

She received short whirlpool sessions daily, followed by debridement of the small, scattered, open wounds around the skin closure. Silvadene was used on the open areas, which were then covered with telfa dressings. The wounds healed quickly without complication.

Range of motion was recorded. The passive range of motion was severely limited at the shoulder, due to pain and the placement of the rod that stabilized the

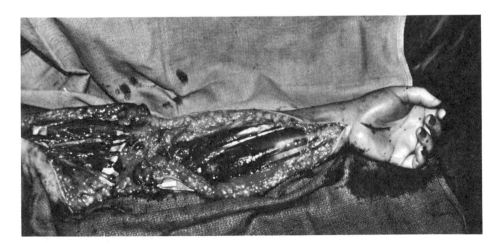

Fig. 5-4. Volar view. Note repaired structures proximal to the elbow. Forearm fasciotomy and carpal tunnel release performed to decrease pressure from edema in the forearm and wrist compartments. (Courtesy of William Shaw, MD, and Stephen Colen, MD.)

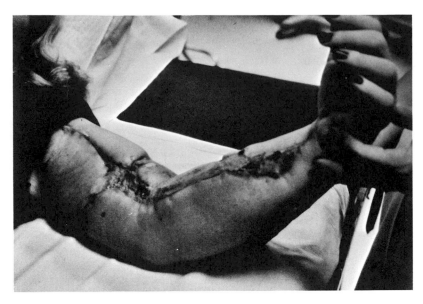

Fig. 5-5.   Patient's first day of therapy. Note edema, elbow flexion contracture, and healing graft on volar aspect of the entire extremity.

humeral fracture. She had an elbow flexion contracture, and her long finger flexors were tight due to the scar on the volar aspect of the wrist, which resulted in limited wrist and finger extension. The metacarpophalangeal joints were limited in flexion, due to the edema on the dorsum of the hand.

Mobilization of all joints was started with good stabilization to avoid movement at the fracture sites. A splint was fabricated to serially stretch the elbow and position the wrist in extension, the MCP joints in flexion, and the IPs extended. Although there was marked flexor tendon tightness, we positioned the hand in the functional position until edema subsided, to overcome the possible shortening of the collateral ligaments that would occur if the MCP joints were to be positioned in extension. The full arm and hand splint was worn overnight. During the day, she wore a wrist control splint with MCP finger flexion saddles attached to an outrigger to increase MCP flexion.

Active range of motion was severely limited, with only poor muscle grades at the shoulder and trace elbow flexion. All other distal musculature was zero. Active range of motion exercises were started in the supine position. The counterbalance sling was used to encourage active assistive movement of the shoulder. Once the patient gained relatively pain free shoulder motion in the counterbalance, she was fitted with a dorsal wrist extension splint with a vertical holder. Adaptive devices fitted into the vertical holder enabled her to use her available shoulder range of motion for specific tasks, i.e., painting. Biofeedback was initiated to encourage active contraction of the biceps.

An early ADL evaluation was completed, as the patient lived alone and had a strong desire to be completely independent. The left replanted extremity was her

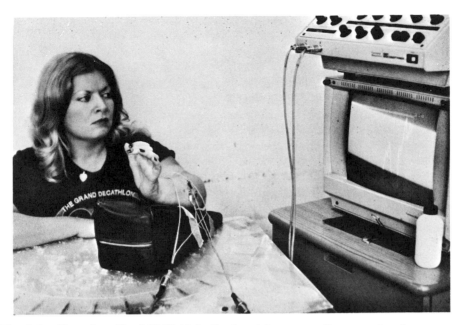

Fig. 5-6. Therapist utilized EMG biofeedback training as an adjunct to other therapy techniques, to aid in the muscle re-education of this patient's extremity.

dominant arm, thus requiring dominance retraining as well as instruction in one-handed activities. A homemaking evaluation and subsequent training were initiated.

As shoulder strength increased to the Fair plus-Good minus range, and innervation progressed to both the triceps and biceps, the table-top balanced forearm orthosis replaced the counterbalance sling for functional retraining. With the distal joints stabilized in the dorsal wrist extension splint, this patient was able to write with the pencil positioned in the vertical holder.

As the triceps became stronger, the patient began to contract the biceps and triceps together whenever active movement was initiated. Due to poor sensation, she had a difficult time isolating each motion. As a result, both movements were inefficient. Biofeedback was used to break this pattern. Electrodes were placed over the biceps and triceps. Muscle and EMG activity were displayed simultaneously on a video screen as two distinct traces. The patient quickly learned to differentiate the two movements and achieved greater active range of motion in both flexion and extension.

Simultaneous innervation of the wrist extensors and flexors at 3 months post-replantation also necessitated biofeedback retraining (Fig. 5-6). The gradual increase in stability at the wrist eventually eliminated the need for the dorsal wrist extension splint for functional activities. A C-clip was used with the vertical holder, which allowed the patient to perform activities despite lack of finger motion (Fig. 5-7).

Extrinsic finger and thumb musculature became palpable at 4 months post-

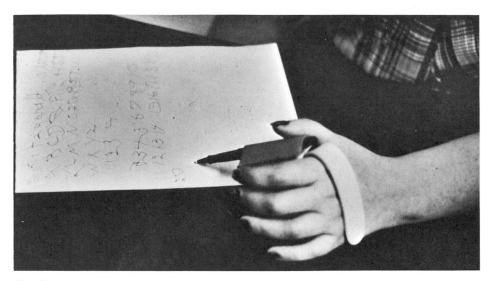

Fig. 5-7. When patient achieved Fair plus wrist extension prior to achieving functional grasp, a C-clip with pen inserted into a vertical holder attachment was utilized to practice writing and as an activity to improve endurance of the wrist extensors.

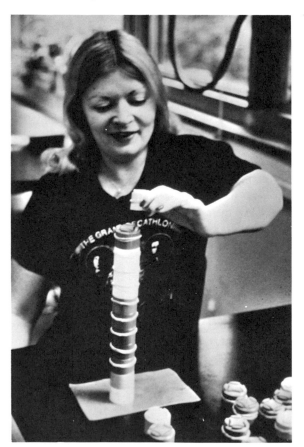

Fig. 5-8. As finger flexors became reinnervated, activities that stressed coordinated arm placement utilizing functional prehension patterns were emphasized.

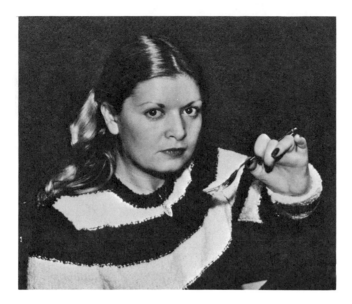

Fig. 5-9.   Patient able to feed herself with minor adjustment of the fork to compensate for limited supination.

replantation. As strength improved, activity selection was aimed at strengthening and improving coordination of prehension patterns (Fig. 5-8). Initially, a short opponens with a lumbrical bar splint was used for thumb positioning and to prevent clawing due to lack of intrinsic musculature. Intrinsic activity was noted at 17 months post-replantation.

During the course of her rehabilitation, the patient required two subsequent surgical procedures. The rod was removed from the forearm after union was complete and the grafted area on the forearm was closed cosmetically. Bone grafting to stabilize the humeral fracture was necessary, after a 1-year trial of electrical stimulation to the fracture site was unsuccessful in promoting adequate callus formation and union. The non-union of the humeral fracture delayed her discharge from therapy. The surgeon wanted to obtain maximum function in the arm prior to surgery, as she would have to be immobilized after the bone grafting. Once the bone graft was well healed, the patient was started on an intense strengthening program, which had been contraindicated while the upper arm was unstable.

A follow-up visit 3 years post-replantation reveals the following status: The patient is enrolled in college with a goal of becoming an occupational therapist. Passive range of motion is minimally limited at the shoulder, elbow, and forearm. She has good plus shoulder strength, good minus elbow strength, poor to fair forearm motion, good extrinsic finger flexors and extensors, and poor intrinsic musculature. Gross grasp measures 3 pounds. She utilizes mainly a lateral pinch for prehension and a gross grip for grasping. (Fig. 5-9). She has protective sensation throughout the arm, but no fine discrimative ability.

CASE STUDY 2

The patient was a 30-year-old male, status post closed oblique fracture of the proximal phalanx digit 3 and replantation of digit 2 at the proximal phalanx of the right dominant hand. The injury occurred when the patient caught his hand in a machine at work. Past medical history showed no contraindications for replantation.

A closed reduction was accomplished with digit 3. Digit 2 sustained a relatively clean cut around the finger just distal to the MCP joint. The fracture was fixated with cross K-wires. Radial and ulnar digital nerves were repaired. Two venous anastomoses were performed with two vein grafts to repair the digital arteries. The flexor digitorum profundus tendon was repaired. Primary skin closure was accomplished. Upon discharge from the hospital the finger was vascularly intact with good capillary refill, and the wound was healing well. Repeat X-rays showed both fractures to be non-displaced and non-angulated.

After 3 weeks of immobilization, the cast was removed and the patient started therapy. Sutures were in place, cross K-wires were protruding from the skin, and small open areas were present around the replantation site. The wound was debrided following a whirlpool treatment. The patient was issued written instructions in wound care and how to bandage his hand. A protective splint was fabricated, positioning the wrist in neutral, with MCPs flexed and IPs extended. Written instructions on care, wearing time, and precautions were reviewed and issued to the patient. Whirlpools and debridement were continued until the wounds were healed. The wrist, thumb, and digits 3 through 5 were stiff from being casted, so joint mobilization was begun and active ROM exercises were taught to the patient, to be carried out at home. Exacting stabilization was utilized during gentle grade I mobilization of MCP, PIP, and DIP joints of digit 3. Minimal active movement was noted at the digit 3 PIP. Gentle active movement was encouraged at this joint.

During the fourth week post-replantation, the pin was removed from digit 2, following an X-ray to determine the extent of bony healing. Active range of motion measures were taken, and gentle AROM, as well as grade I mobilization with exacting stabilization, was begun at the PIP and DIP joints of digit 2. Light prehension activities were begun, alternating each digit with the thumb to encourage AROM.

At 5 weeks post-replantation, the wounds were healed. Edema was evaluated and a coban wrap issued to decrease the edema in digits 2 and 3, as well as an isotoner glove to be worn overnight to decrease the minimal edema present in the entire hand. Passive range of motion was evaluated, and gentle PROM exercises were begun. A flexion assist splint was fabricated to increase passive flexion of all the joints of digits 2 and 3. Bunnell blocks to increase active PIP flexion of digits 2 and 3 were also fabricated. An ADL evaluation revealed that the patient had difficulty eating and cutting meat with the involved hand, so built-up handled utensils were issued to encourage the patient to begin using the impaired hand. He had difficulty with many bilateral tasks, and was instructed as to how he could use what function he had in the involved hand to complete these tasks. Writing practice was begun to further encourage functional use.

Once edema had subsided somewhat, a sensory evaluation was completed, which revealed moving touch to be grossly intact but localization to be absent. Hot-cold and deep touch were absent, rendering digit 2 essentially anesthetic. Sensation elsewhere in the hand was intact.

At approximately 6 weeks post-replantation, the fracture sites were healed sufficiently to withstand stress. The hand function test and manual muscle test were administered, as well as dynamometer and pinch meter readings to assess strength. More aggressive passive stretching was tolerated, and resistive hand strengthening exercises were begun. MCP joint ROM was now normal in digits 2 and 3, so an MCP block was added to the dynamic flexion splint so that the flexion forces would be concentrated at the PIP joints and DIP joints. Heavy resistive activities were gradually added, particularly those involving tool use, as this was part of his job requirement. He was being followed by a vocational counselor throughout this outpatient status and until he returned to work.

At the time of discharge, gross grasp measured 36 lb, palmar pinch 5 lb, and lateral pinch 8 lb. Sensation improved significantly, with 7 mm of moving two-point discrimiation on the radial and ulnar aspects of digit 2. Active range of motion was normal throughout the hand, with the exception of the digit 2 PIP joint, which measured 15 to 60° of motion and the digit 3 PIP joint which measured 0 to 95°.

A follow-up evaluation 1 ½ years post-replantation reveals the following status: PROM of digit 2 PIP joint improved to 5 to 80°, AROM 5 to 70°. PROM of digit 3 PIP joint measures 0 to 100° and AROM 0 to 90° (Fig. 5-10, 11). Gross grasp is now 52 lb, compared to 75 lb on the left; palmar pinch is 25 lb, and lateral pinch is 20 lb. Palmar and lateral pinch are now equal to that of the left hand. Sensation shows significant improvement and is now considered normal, with 3 mm of moving two-point discrimination in the autonomous zones of the digital nerves to digit 2 and 5 mm of static two-point discrimination. The patient is independent in activities of daily living, i.e., dressing, eating, hygiene, and a variety of simple home management tasks. He cannot sustain an activity that requires power gripping or heavy resistance, due to pain in the involved digits (Fig. 5-12). As a result, although he has returned to work, his job has been modified to eliminate these types of tasks. The patient experiences hypersensitivity to cold, although he appears to be less sensitive 1 ½ years post-replantation than he was upon discharge from an active therapy program.

LONG-TERM PROBLEMS

The major long-term problems encountered when treating the replantation patients are unfavorable adhesion formation, resulting in stiff joints, and flexor tendon adherence. Often, by the time the pins are out the tendons have already adhered. We then work toward full passive mobility in preparation for a tenolysis or two-stage tendon reconstruction. It deserves mention that we have not seen good results following two-stage tendon reconstruction with the replantation population.

Excessive edema and post-surgical complications that delay the initiation of early

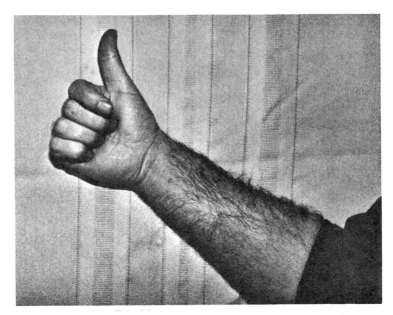

Fig. 5-10.　18 months post-replantation—lacks 5° active proximal interphalangeal joint extension of digit 2.

therapy, such as infection, lead to a higher incidence of stiff joints. If the stiffness cannot be overcome within the late therapy phases, then capsulotomies are performed.

With replantations at the level of the proximal phalanx, we find that the patient seldom achieves a good flexion arc at the PIP joint. If there is a reasonably good

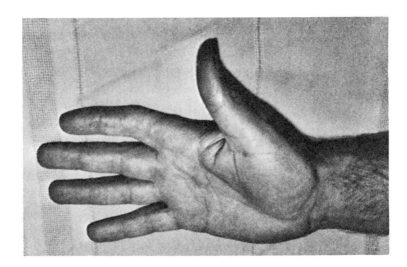

Fig. 5-11.　18 months post-replantation—lacks 30° active proximal interphalangeal joint flexion of digit 2.

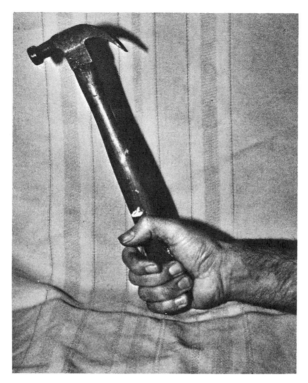

Fig. 5-12.   18 months post-replantation—gross grasp sufficient to hold a hammer.

chance of nerve regeneration and the replant is of the second or third digit, we feel that the proximal interphalangeal joint should be fused in a position of flexion to produce a stable pinch. An unstable, anesthetic digit only gets in the way and is at risk for injury.

Non-unions are seldom a problem, but they occur mainly when the fracture is in close proximity to a joint or when infection necessitates early pin removal. Bone grafting may be necessary to stabilize the fracture. Prolonged immobilization due to delayed bony union makes achievement of joint mobility and tendon gliding difficult and questionable.

The majority of our patients do achieve protective sensation, and a smaller number achieve discriminative ability in their fingers. If sensation has failed to progress, neuroloysis or nerve grafting will be necessary. Secondary surgeries are delayed until the patient's active and passive movement has plateaued, since secondary immobilization will cause additional stiffness.

With upper arm replantations, we have observed intrinsic hand musculature reinnervation, but only of trace or poor strength. Protective sensation is likely; however, discriminative ability is lacking.

Cold intolerance is experienced by all of our patients to greater or lesser degrees, but usually subsides with time. We suggest that the patient use maximum protection when exposed to cold temperatures. Battery operated hunting mittens are recommended for severe cases.

REFERENCES

1. Malt RA, McKahn C: Replantation of severed limbs. JAMA 189:716, 1964
2. Macleod MB, O'Brien BM, Morrison WA: Digital replantation clinical experiences. Clin Orthop 133: 27, 1978
3. Morrison WA, O'Brien B, MacLeod AM: Evaluation of digital replantation—a review of 100 cases. Orthop Clin North Am 8:2, 1977
4. O'Brien B: Replantation surgery. Clin Plast Sur 1(3):405 1974
5. Urbaniak JR: P. 811. In Green DP (ed): Replantation in Operative Hand Surgery. Churchill Livingsone, New York, 1982
6. Weiland AJ, Villarreal-Rios A, Kleinert HE et al: Replantation of digits and hands: Analysis of surgical techniques and functional results in 71 patients with 86 replantations. J Hand Surg 2:1, 1977
7. Beasley RW: Hand Injuries. WB Saunders, Philadelphia, 1981
8. Wang S, Young K, Wei J: Replantation of severed limbs—Clinical analysis of ninety one cases. J Hand Surg 6:311, 1981
9. Wilson CS, Alpert BC, Bunke HJ, Gordon L: Replantation of the upper extremity. Clin Plast Surg 10:85, 1983
10. Dellon AL: Evaluation of Sensibility and Re-education of Sensation in the Hand. Williams & Wilkins, Baltimore, 1981
11. Evans D: The healing process at cellular level: A review. Physiotherapy 66: 1980
12. Madden JW: Wound healing: The biological basis of hand surgery. In Hunter, Schneider, Mackin, Bell (eds): Rehabilitation of the Hand. CV Mosby Co, St Louis, 1978
13. Weeks PM, Wray RC: Management of Acute Hand Injuries: A Biological Approach. CV Mosby Co, St Louis, 1978
14. Chen ZW, Meyer UE, Kleinert HE: Present indications and contraindications for replantation as reflected by long-term functional results. Orthop Clin North Am, 3:849, 1981
15. Mackin EJ, Maiorano L: Postoperative therapy following staged tendon reconstruction. In Hunter, Schneider, Mackin, Bell (eds): Rehabilitation of the Hand. CV Mosby Co, St Louis, 1978
16. Nissenbaumm M: Early care of flexor tendon injuries, application of principles of tendon healing and early motion, In Hunter, Schneider, Mackin, Bell (eds): Rehabilitation of the Hand. CV Mosby Co, St Louis, 1978
17. Prendergast K: Therapists' management of a mutilated hand. In Hunter, Schneider, Mackin, Bell (eds): Rehabilitation of the Hand. CV Mosby Co, St Louis, 1978
18. Kilgore ES, Grahan WP: The Hand: Surgical and Nonsurgical Management. Lea & Febiger, Philadelphia, 1977
19. Matsen FA, Wyss CP, Simmons CW: The effects of compression and elevation on the circulation to the skin of the hand as reflected by transcutaneous PO_2. Plast Reconstr Surg 69:86, 1982
20. Evans EB, Eggers GWN, Butler JK, Blumel J: Experimental immobilization and remobilization of the rat knee joints. J Bone Joint Surg 42-A:737, 1980
21. Rubak JM, Poussa M, Ritsila V: Effects of joint motion on the repair of articular cartilage with free periosteal grafts. Acta Orthop Scand 53:187, 1982
22. Salter RB, Simmonds DF, Malcolm BW et al: The effects of continuous passive motion on the healing of articular cartilage defects. J Bone Joint Surg 57-A:570, 1975
23. Akeson A, Mechanic G, Woo S et al: Collagen cross-linking alterations in joint contractures: changes in the reducible cross-links in periarticular connective tissue collagen after nine weeks of immobilization. Connect Tissue Res, 5:15, 1977

6 | The Therapist's Role in Finger Joint Arthroplasty

Donald G. Shurr

Theoretically, prosthetic replacement of the abnormal joint would supply the movement of an arthroplasty and the stability of a fusion. This attractive theory has not yet been translated into practical fact. No prosthesis exists which can approach the stability and versatility of a normal joint. All mechanical devices so far produced are inadequate substitutes and most have severe drawbacks.

—Dr. Adrian E. Flatt, 1962*

The role of the therapist in the treatment of finger joint replacement arthroplasty may vary, but most authors agree that the postoperative program is equal in importance to the surgical procedure. Other authors believe that patients who are unwilling or unable to complete the postoperative therapy sessions will not enjoy a successful result, and surgery should be delayed or postponed until those arrangements can be made.

HISTORICAL PERSPECTIVE

The role of the therapist in the care of patients with replacement arthroplasty is evolving with time. Brannon and Klein[1] in 1959 referred to the need for postoperative, early, active, and graduated exercise to be done until maximum function was attained. No mention was made of the necessity for any therapist, and presumably the surgeon taught the exercises and they were done by the patient without supervision. This phi-

---

*Reprinted with permission from Journal of Bone and Joint Surgery 54A(3):435, 1972.

losophy contrasts with entire chapters of books devoted to the postoperative program for a particular type of device, such as Leonard's[2] chapter dealing with the Swanson spacer.

The change in postoperative philosophy, or rather the development of a rationale of postoperative care, can be related to the increased awareness of the normal response to healing and the knowledge of this information within the hand surgery community. Madden and DeVore[3] spoke to this point in their fine work published in 1977.

As more information about healing and the biomechanical effects that forces and joints have on the healing process become available, changes in postoperative care will need to be made.

Although joint arthroplasty, and specifically replacement joint arthroplasty, may be indicated for many types of patients with varying pathologies, a large percentage of the current surgical indications is reconstruction of the rheumatoid hand. Brannon and Klein first replaced joints in otherwise normal military personnel. Flatt[4] spoke of the unrealistic expectation for replacement arthroplasty, citing his belief that only in otherwise unsalvable hands should artificial joints be placed. Recently, varying success has been reported using replacement arthroplasty for normal patients having abnormal finger joints. Although no agreement appears imminent as to which problems replacement arthroplasty will best solve, the postoperative care of such patients should continue to be developed, changed, and explained using the scientific process. Accountability for the postoperative role of the therapist should be measured to allow careful analysis of the postoperative outcomes, in order to improve those portions of the overall program needing change, while not changing others that appear sound.

For the purposes of this chapter, the studies reviewed and referenced, unless otherwise stated, relate to patients having rheumatoid arthritis, since these represent the largest group. Appropriate reference will be made to the few reports that deal with replacement arthroplasty in other than patients with rheumatoid arthritis.

Although artificial joints have been surgically placed in many joints of the wrist and hand, this chapter concerns the thumb carpometacarpal (CMC), the finger metacarpophalangeal (MCP), and the finger proximal interphalangeal (PIP) joints. The distal interphalangeal (DIP) joint is mentioned and referenced simply for completeness.

THERAPIST OR THERAPIST

Chronologically, the first therapist was undoubtedly the surgeon, as early postoperative care of hand problems was provided directly by the surgeon. Gradually, nurses accepted a greater role in the postoperative care of hands. Polio and world wars opened the way for both physical and occupational therapists to enter the arena of hand therapy. Medical specialization and specifically the hand surgeon gave birth to the concept of a hand therapist. The hand therapist represents a meld of usually physical or occupational therapists specifically dealing with hand patients and hand problems. Hand therapists deal with the entire group of hand problems and rehabilitation, providing evaluation and treatment, often in an outpatient, free-standing facility. The American Society of Hand Therapists, established in 1977, acknowledges the creativity and the need for further development of such a professional service.

GENERATIONS OF IMPLANTS

First Generation

The first generation of finger joint implant was that of a solid, stainless steel, single-axis hinge type joint (Fig. 6-1). Using the early experience of Brannon and Klein, Flatt modified the block and hinge by adding two prongs to the stems of the prosthesis, in an effort to better control rotation.

Second Generation

The second generation represents the all plastic concept (Fig. 6-2). The best-known examples of the second generation are the Swanson and the Niebauer types. The Swanson is a one-piece flexible implant. A capsule of scar forms around the implant, but the implant remains free to glide in the joint cavity.

The Niebauer, now marketed as the Sutter, is also made of medical-grade silicone rubber, but employs a block design and is impregnated with dacron, used to strengthen the hinge. Additionally, the Niebauer employs a dacron cover and sutures, which are thought to be responsible for both early and long-term fixation. Sutures tied to bone maintain it for 6 weeks, until tissue growth restrains it within the medullary canal.

Third Generation

The third generation consists of a two-piece articulated prosthesis made from two dissimilar materials. High-density polyethylene comprises the metacarpal component, and the phalangeal component is made from stainless steel. All third generation prostheses require cement for implantation. The Schultz and the Steffe are representative of the third generation (Fig. 6-3).

Newer Designs and Materials

Clinical experience with these three generations of designs and materials indicates that problems remain. Less constrained designs, combined with newer materials, have allowed the introduction of two new devices: the Heiple and the Mayo pyrolytic carbon MCP prostheses.

The Heiple Mark I and Mark II, Biomeric total joint has reportedly been used in the replacement arthroplasty of over 200 MCP joints. A sample of Mark I types has been followed for up to 3.5 years. The Mark II, used in 54 joints, has been followed for up to 1 year. Results are mixed; pain relief and short-term realignment of joints is accomplished. Complications of fracture, infection, and recurrent joint positions remain problems of this new variety of implant.

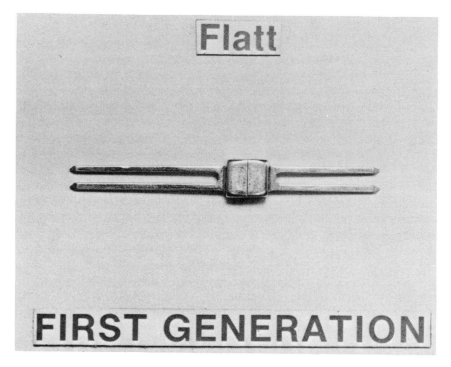

Fig. 6-1.   The First Generation: A Flatt Prosthesis.

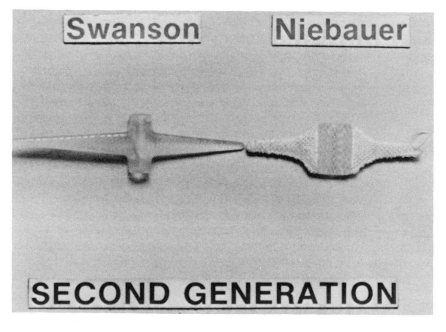

Fig. 6-2.   The Second Generation: A Swanson Spacer and the Niebauer marketed by Cutter.

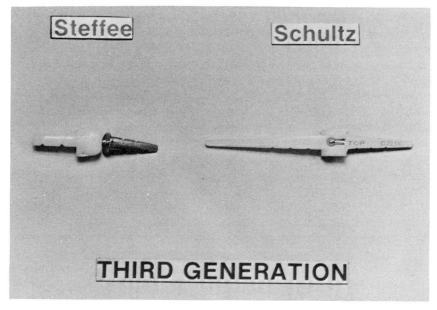

Fig. 6-3.   The Third Generation: A Steffee and a Schultz, both requiring cement for fixation.

The Heiple implant contains titanium stems, with a curvilinear plane bonded to an elastomeric polyolefin midsection, hinged on a solid rod. The stems require cement for fixation. Since the rod is continuous, flexion of the implant takes place in the middle.

Pyrolitic carbons have been used in many implants placed elsewhere than the hand. Dentists use such carbons for facial implants. Hip prostheses utilize pyrolitic carbons to eliminate the use of bone cement, thought to strengthen the implant-bone interface.

Robert D. Beckenbaugh, MD, from the Mayo Clinic, is using the non-cemented, non-constrained device. The use of the implant allows less bone resection, and the non-constrained design is thought to prevent or lessen loosening. Early results identify the importance of proper balancing of the fingers in order to reduce the tendency for recurrent problems.

Pyrolysis refers to the decomposition of organic substances under the influence of a rise in temperature. Pyrolite carbon is a turbostatic pyrolytic carbon produced by the decomposition of a hydrocarbon gas at 1,400°C, a temperature that is low compared to the melting point of carbon. Pyrolite carbon is deposited as a thick coating (1 mm) on a graphite substrate. The articulating surfaces of the implants are polished. Tissue fixation areas remain on the stems, as deposited, which provides a rough surface for tissue ingrowth.

Postoperative care using both types of implants is quite similar to that used with the second generation types. Initially, the pyrolitic carbons were thought to subluxate and, as a result, were maintained in extension for 3 weeks. Currently, a program similar to that used with conventional silastic spacers is utilized, involving early motion and dynamic splints for extension, begun 5 to 7 days postoperatively. A combination

Table 6-1. Carpometacarpal Patient Data

Authors	Patients	Thumbs	Women	Men	Rheumatoid Arthritis	Degenerative Joint Disease
Ashworth[7]	42	49	35	7	3	39
Ferlic[9]	11	11	9	2	0	11
Kessler[8b]	19	19	14	5	0	19
Poppen[8]	15	17	12	3	4	11
Swanson[8a]	38	46	32	6	11	27
Totals	125	142	102	23	18 (14.4%)	107 (85.6%)

of night resting splints and dynamic day splints continues for 3 months postoperatively.

CARPOMETACARPAL JOINT ARTHROPLASTY

Although the silastic implant used for carpometacarpal (CMC) joint replacement arthroplasty resembles the second generation MCP silicone rubber type, its purpose and, therefore, the design are much different. Replacement arthroplasty of the saddle joint of the thumb is often done for degenerative disease in otherwise normal individuals. Although the procedure may be indicated in people with rheumatoid disease, Table 6-1 indicates that 85.6 percent of the CMC joints replaced were for degenerative joint disease, while only 14.4 percent were rheumatoid arthritis.

Indications

The surgical indications for replacement arthroplasty of the CMC joint are uniform: pain and joint instability. Since the expected outcome is for a stable, pain-free joint, the postoperative care of these patients is different from that for other types of replacement arthroplasty.

Postoperative Management

Following surgery, the thumb is placed in a plaster cast extending above the wrist. Swanson prefers to keep the first and second metacarpal in 40 to 60° of palmar abduction. Swanson also prefers a scaphoid forearm cast for 3 to 4 days to apply pressure to the metacarpals, not the phalanges. Ashworth reports using a large compression dressing and a volar plaster splint to keep the thumb abducted. This is removed 10 days postoperatively, and a thumb spica cast is applied for 4 to 5 weeks. Swanson reports using a short arm cast 4 to 6 weeks following the removal of the initial cast. Poppen reports using a plaster cast above the wrist for 4 to 6 weeks to allow healing and/or scarring to occur.

Most authors agree that active range of motion exercises to tolerance may be started following cast removal. Full, pain-free motion is possible by the end of 3 months. Swanson reports full, unguarded motion to be indicated by 6 to 10 weeks postoperatively.

Postoperative Results

Results of these series typically report range of motion, pain, and grip strength. Poppen reports a follow-up average for radial abduction of the first and second metacarpals to be 18.5°. Ashworth reported ratings for 49 patients, averaging 31 months follow-up. Forty of 49 rated their results to be excellent, which assumed equal or greater abduction and grip strength, and no pain, when compared with the normal thumb CMC joint.

Pain was relieved in 12 of 15 patients, according to Poppen. At an average follow-up of 20 months, Ferlic reported that all patients (11) were satisfied following the procedure, principally because of pain relief. Swanson reported that pain was completely relieved in all 46 cases.

Strength was usually reported as pinch and grip, both requiring a stable thumb CMC joint. Swanson reported an average of 2.3 kg of pinch and 4.5 kg of grip increase gained following surgery. Pinch ranged from 2.3 to 4.5 kg for females and 6.8 to 9.1 for males. Grip ranged from 13.1 to 18.0 kg for females and 41.9 to 46.5 kg for males. Ferlic reported that strength improved in 5 of 11 cases, when comparing preoperative and postoperative data. Poppen reported that postoperative pinch was equal to or greater than preoperative pinch in 9 of 14 cases. Grip increased in 13 of 14 cases; the one exception had severe rheumatoid arthritis.

Complications

One cause of failure in this procedure is prosthetic joint subluxation or dislocation, which produces a lack of joint stability. Poppen reported 6 cases of subluxation, 2 of which were complete, in his series of 17. Swanson reported 8 radial subluxation complications in his series of 46, most of which could be attributed to either the surgical procedure or the design of the prosthesis. Table 6-2 denotes the data compiled from five published series.

Summary

Replacement arthroplasty for the CMC joint provides pain relief and stability following surgery. Some authors believe it does not provide near normal strength, but most agree that it does allow normal daily activities and does relieve pain.

LONG-TERM FOLLOW-UP USING FIRST GENERATION IMPLANTS

Development of Metallic Hinged Prostheses

In 1940, Burman[10] implanted inert foreign material into finger joints. Using vitallium caps, he attempted to resurface three interphalangeal (IP) joints of patients with traumatic injury. Brannon and Klein reported on a total joint excision with metallic replacement in 1959, using a one-piece, single-axis steel prosthesis. Brannon and Klein

Table 6-2. Complications Reported Following CMC Replacement

Author[a]	Operations	Fractures	Dislocations
Ashworth[7]	49	2	0
Ferlic[9]	11	0	0
Kessler[8b]	41	0	0
Poppen[8]	17	0	6
Swanson[8a]	46	0	8
Total	164	2	14

felt that the procedure was contraindicated in the clinical presence of any active inflammatory, rheumatic, or bacterial processes, using active military personnel with traumatic conditions as their subjects. Flatt, on the other hand, felt that the procedure should be restricted to otherwise unsalvable hands, as a last resort, using them entirely on people having rheumatoid arthritis. Brannon and Klein recognized the potential problem with rotational instability, adding a triangular intramedullary stem. Flatt changed the triangular stem to two prongs, in an effort to control rotation.

Results

The results using Brannon and Klein's steel prosthesis were reported in 14 patients, 12 of whom were followed for 10 to 39 months. Most retained a functional, pain-free range of motion. Stability of the joints was satisfactory. By definition, a satisfactory result measured 50° of PIP motion, minimal or no symptoms, work performance without complaint, and some x-ray evidence of migration of the prosthesis in the bone. The authors not only recognized this problem, but were concerned about it, adding a nail through the cortices and the stem in an effort to control it. Overall results numbered 10 cases at least satisfactory in follow-up. Pain relief was achieved.

Flatt[11] reported after 14 years, using 242 metallic prostheses in 84 patients with rheumatoid arthritis between 1957 and 1971. 167 were MCP and 75 were PIP. Average follow-up time was 6.2 years. Flatt reported active range of motion of the MCP joint at follow-up to be 16° at 0 to 7 months; 25° at 8 months to 5 years; 16° at 5 to 14 years. Flatt proposed that this decrease in active range of motion was due largely to periarticular fibrosis.

POSTOPERATIVE MANAGEMENT—FIRST GENERATION

Postoperative care of these metallic joints was not aggressive in today's terms. The hand was placed in a bulky dressing with dorsal compression and elevated for 3 days. Following wound inspection, the joints were immobilized in extension for 2 weeks. Sutures were then removed and splints re-applied. It was at 4 weeks postoperatively that gentle motion was started. The role of the therapist at this point was in preoperative evaluation and postoperative follow-up, attempting to gain motion from 4 weeks on.

Dryer[12] et al. reported on 29 patients with Flatt PIP joints. Active PIP range of motion varied from 20° in 0 to 3.5 years follow-up, to 11° in joints followed for longer than 9.6 years, demonstrating a gradual decrease in average range of motion over time. Average grip strength and key grip measurements also decreased with time. Most patients reported pain relief and a general positive feeling about their procedures. Most would submit to the same procedures again if it were necessary. Many of the patients volunteered that stability was more important than flexibility.

Blair, Shurr, and Buckwalter[13] reported on 43 patients having metallic Flatt MCP prosthetic implants. All had rheumatoid arthritis and were followed for an average of 11.5 years. Average range of motion was 24°, with a range of 0 to 95°. Recurrent deviation occurred in 58 percent of the cases.

Complications

Although patient satisfaction was reported to be high, poor tolerance of metal in bone has largely reduced the use of metallic prostheses. Progressive absorption of bone around metal has rendered some joints totally motionless. Girzadas and Clayton[14] commented on the inevitable bone resorption, calling it "by far the most serious complication." The unpredictable clinical results with the Flatt prosthesis may be considered an objection to its use.

THE SECOND GENERATION: THE ALL PLASTIC SPACER CONCEPT

Silicones, or polydimethylsiloxanes, comprise a variety of implantable medical devices. The finger joint spacer is an example of such an application used because of high biological compatibility. These silicones, which have been commercially available since the early 1940s, were extensively tested through the 1950s, and became the treatment of choice for shunts in hydrocephalus.

The formulations of "soft, medium, and firm" silicones have generally been referred to as "medical grade silicone elastomeres," and comprise the materials of the second generation spacers for finger joints.

Although many researchers have worked with plastic finger joints, Dr. A. B. Swanson,[15] an orthopedist from Grand Rapids, Michigan, pioneered the use of these materials in a wide variety of surgical, implantable devices, the best-known of which is the finger joint of the Swanson design.

Any discussion of silicone rubber spacers would be incomplete without mention of the "encapsulation process." According to Swanson, "The implant glides 1 or 2 mm in the intramedullary canals on flexion and extension movements. Gliding allows a greater range of motion to occur and permits the implant to find the best position with respect to the axis of rotation of the joint."

According to Madden, DeVore, and Arem, the encapsulation process appears, by histologic criteria, to be complete by 6 to 8 weeks postoperatively. The spacers are surrounded by a scar capsule composed of moderately thick collagen bundles and a small number of fibroblasts. However, according to Madden, clinical observation demonstrates progressive change of shape with time. Since animal experimentation clearly demonstrates changes and metabolic activity in a maturing scar, a rationale can be developed to care for the dynamic situation following implant arthroplasty.

The reader is advised of the fine contribution made by Madden to the rationale for effective splinting used following replacement arthroplasty. Anyone seeking to treat any number of these patients should make the Madden article a *must* prior to program implementation.

Candidates for Surgery

As stated by Mannerfelt,[16] the goals of replacement arthroplasty may be varied and often represent a combination of objectives which may vary from one hand to the other. Severe joint and soft tissue contractures may require motion to achieve function, whereas the totally flail joint may require joint stability. Progressive ulnar deviation leads to a hand without prehension, demanding a complete assessment of the proposed repositioning of the fingers and consideration of the condition and position of the thumb. Many surgical candidates have severe pain, which leads them to seek surgery. Generally, a progressive inability to function at a suitable level constitutes the indication for surgical reconstruction of finger joints.

The relevant literature records two basic designs: one by Swanson and marketed by Dow Corning; the other design by Niebauer, more recently marketed by Sutter. Most clinical studies of these two designs feature a relatively short follow-up and attempt to quantify a positive postoperative result. Most results report clinical use with patients having rheumatoid arthritis. More recently, the results feature a plea for a complete postoperative program as a prerequisite to admittance to the program, something the early studies failed to recognize. Often, reports of clinical trials represent a combination of philosophies and practices, making each contribution difficult to separate and impossible to evaluate.

The Niebauer-Sutter silicone rubber–Dacron-covered prosthesis employs a biconcave hinge with Dacron weave around each stem. The Dacron weave becomes fixed inside the medullary canals, achieving fixation. Motion occurs about the flexible stem, and may be extremely variable from one unit to another.

The Axes of Rotation

Much has been written concerning the location of the axis of rotation of the MCP joint in the finger. Flatt describes the joint as one with a transverse axis of flexion and extension, as well as radial and ulnar deviation. Schultz, Swanson, and Walker[17] believe that the center is not fixed and moves as the finger joint moves. Youm[18] states that movement of the MCP joint in either flexion-extension or radial-ulnar deviation occurs about a fixed center located near the head of the metacarpal. Any prosthetic replacement should locate its axis of rotation near that anatomical point. Variations in the location of the center of rotation, usually in the dorsal direction, may lead to an imbalance in favor of the flexion movement, producing an extensor lag.

According to Gillespie,[19] the biomechanical behavior of commercially available devices with respect to center of rotation in flexion-extension and radial-ulnar deviation vary widely, and none duplicate the normal MCP joint. There is also variation upon repeated tests with the same prosthesis or spacer, and variation between two devices of the same design and material. The readers would be well advised to read the entire article by Gillespie for an excellent review of mechanics related to finger joints.

VARIABLES AFFECTING POSTOPERATIVE RESULTS

Since controlled, prospective studies of rheumatoid hand reconstruction are difficult, if not impossible, to complete, most studies report retrospective clinical results at 1 to 5 years post-surgery. According to Madden, successful results using all plastic, second generation type implants depend on (1) proper patient selection, (2) adequate operative technique, and (3) careful postoperative management. The hand therapist may play an important role in proper patient selection and is the catalyst which ensures proper postoperative management. Many therapists treat potential arthroplasty patients with conservative care for hand problems as the disease progresses, involving the wrists, MCPs, and PIPs. This experience brings a valuable contribution to the ultimate decision of which procedure is indicated and when it should be performed. Surgeons rely on the expertise and judgment of the hand therapist when evaluating: (1) the functional limitations of each patient, (2) the functional changes as the disease progresses or the patient responds to treatment, (3) the expectations of the patient, and (4) the support available in the patient's household and community.

MCP POSTOPERATIVE CARE

The recommended postoperative care following finger joint arthroplasty began rather conservatively. Flatt and Niebauer both recommended immobilization followed by exercise. Flatt[20] recommended 8 to 10 days of splinting in extension, with alternating current to the extensors. Niebauer[21] recommended splinting the MCP joints in extension for 3 to 4 weeks, followed by active exercise. Using the Niebauer device, Urbaniak[22] recommended that the joints be splinted in full extension, with motion begun at 14 to 21 days postoperatively. He stated that there is no valid correlation between when motion is begun and the eventual outcome in range of motion. He stated that since fixation requires 2 to 3 weeks, motion should not start until then. A dorsal outrigger to maintain the MCP joints in extension and slight radial deviation is employed at 14 to 21 days and continued for 3 to 4 months. The preoperative evaluation done by the hand therapist contributes to the timing of the surgical procedures and the expectations of the patient at follow-up. Splinting is generally thought best accomplished early, begun 3 to 5 days postoperatively and continued until the joints are stable, usually at 3 to 4 months. (Fig. 6-4) Well written book chapters and articles on the exact means by which such splints may be accomplished are cited in the reference list and in Chapter 9.

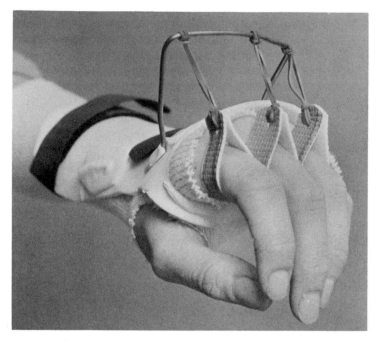

Fig. 6-4.   A dorsal, dynamic extension splint used following MCP implant arthroplasty.

POSTOPERATIVE CARE: THE PIP JOINT

Swanson[23] divides the postoperative care for implant arthroplasty of the proximal interphalangeal joint into three groups: (1) following arthroplasty for stiff PIPs, (2) following arthroplasty for swan-neck deformity, and (3) following arthroplasty for boutonniere deformity.

Arthroplasty Management for Stiff PIP Joint

Following implant arthroplasty without tendon reconstruction for stiff PIPs, active flexion-extension should begin within 3 to 5 days post-surgery. Splints to maintain 0° extension are worn at night for several weeks, depending on the degree of extensor lag. A few degrees of extensor lag should be expected, according to Swanson. Angular deformities may be maintained by taping the aluminum splint to the appropriate side of the finger. No lateral forces affecting the PIP joint should be allowed.

Management for Swan-Neck Deformity

Following implant arthroplasty for swan-neck deformity with tendon reconstruction, the finger is splinted in 10 to 20 degrees of flexion for 10 days. After 10 days, exercises in flexion are begun, being careful to extend only to 10°, so as not to encourage recurrent swan-neck deformity. A palmar lumbrical bar, supporting the MCPs near extension, can assist in isolating motion of the PIPs.

Management for Boutonniere Deformity

Following implant arthroplasty for boutonniere deformity, the motions encouraged are PIP extension and DIP flexion. The extensor mechanism should be protected for 10 days following resolution of postoperative edema, which may last for 3 weeks total. An aluminum splint should immobilize the PIP joint in extension for 3 to 6 weeks, continuing at night for up to 10 weeks. The distal interphalangeal (DIP) joint is allowed to flex.

Active flexion and extension exercises are encouraged using a combination of appropriate blocking techniques described by Bunnell and others, or transverse lumbrical bars or thermoplastic splints.

Swanson states that the responsibility for the postoperative care should be managed by the surgeon and not delegated to another physician.

RESULTS OF CLINICAL STUDIES

Reis and Calnan[24] reported on the use of a polypropylene integral hinger joint used for PIP replacement. In 1969 they stated that the results of PIP were more encouraging than the MCP. They also stated that very early mobilization of the PIP joint serves no purpose and may endanger the deformity correction. They recommended that the joints be immobilized for 3 weeks, until sound healing occurred. Splinting should continue for 3 months.

Strickland[25] reported results of 100 traumatic PIP replacements using spacers of the second generation. At follow-up, 75 percent reportedly were pain free, with an average extensor lag of 20°, and further flexion to 63°, or an arc of 43°. The patient group was followed from 3 months to 4 years, with an average of 7.4 months.

Postoperative care was dependent on the presence of an intact extensor tendon. With extensor tendon intact, motion began at 3 days, with static extension splints alternated with dynamic flexion splints. If the extensor tendon had been reconstructed, extension splints continued for 3 weeks, allowing the tendon to heal. Static extension and dynamic flexion splints were then used.

Dryer, Blair, Shurr and Buckwalter[26] reported on 30 Swanson and 7 Niebauer second generation implants. Follow-up of the Swanson type averaged 4.3 years, and of the Niebauer type 6.2 years. All demonstrated progressive loss of range of motion with time. Active range of motion with Swansons averaged 40° at 0 to 3.5 years and was reduced to 26° at 6.6 to 9.5 years follow-up.

Postoperative care of this group was mixed, but generally entailed 2 weeks of post-surgical immobilization in extension, followed by gentle, active flexion exercise and appropriate extension splints. Clinical fusion of the joint with the implant occurred with all three types (including Flatt). Eight cases of recurrent swan-neck deformity were found in the Swanson types, and three cases of recurrent boutonniere deformity occurred in the Niebauer types.

Given these data, 24 of 29 patients said that they would seek the surgery again in the same situation. All were relieved of PIP joint pain, and 24 of 29 felt that both function and appearance were subjectively improved following the surgery.

POSTOPERATIVE CARE USING THIRD GENERATION IMPLANTS

Using cemented third generation prostheses, motion may be initiated earlier, since medial-lateral support is a product of the prosthetic design. Linscheid[27] reported that splinted, protected motion began between 3 and 21 days postoperatively, usually by the seventh day. Extension splints were used for 2 to 10 weeks. Full, active flexion was discouraged for 3 to 6 weeks. There were no good results in 67 fingers; the problems were usually related to extensor lag or lack of active extension.

OTHER VARIABLES AFFECTING POSTOPERATIVE OUTCOME

Other variables affecting the results of clinical studies are the exacerbations and remissions occurring with a given patient, differing disease expressions among patients, and the evolution of drug therapy. These factors affect the postoperative clinical course and, thus, the clinical results. The evolution of drug therapy is an especially important factor. Over the period of time in which most of the data presented was collected, a wide variety of non-steroid, antiinflammatory drugs (NSAIDS), were created. Many patients took any of a number of these plus aspirin, gold, penicillamine, steroids, methotrexate, and imuran. Since the approach to drug therapy is ever-changing, the clinical results of reported clinical studies using implants are complicated by the use of many drugs. Various new and heretofore uncategorized diseases and mixtures of diseases may have been referred to previously as pure rheumatoid arthritis, whereas they may represent a mixture of collagen vascular diseases not well understood. For these many reasons, predictable outcomes following joint arthroplasty must be presented with guarded optimism.

ISSUES AFFECTING LONG-TERM RESULTS

In addition to the limitations in clinical studies of rheumatoid hand reconstruction already mentioned, the reader should be aware of several remaining issues which concern the results of finger joint arthroplasty.

The issues which remain certainly affect potential clinical outcomes. They involve many processes over which minimal control presently exists. These issues include recurrent ulnar deviation; subluxation and contracture of the joint; durability of the implant itself, including fracture and cold flow seen with polyethelenes; host bone tolerance, including resorption and ectopic bone formation and cement-bone interface problems in third generation cemented prostheses.

Other issues which have been reported will be contrasted within the limits of clin-

Table 6-3. Report of Clinical Studies Using Second Generation Implants

Study	Number of Implants	Fracture (%)	Dislocation (%)	Infection (%)	Recurrent Ulnar deviation	Range of Motion (Degrees) Pre-Op	Range of Motion (Degrees) Post-Op
Swanson	3,409	1	1	1	2	—	4–57
Swanson	358	2	1	1	3	—	3–64
Braun	80	1	0	0	0	—	10–70
Ferlic	165	9	—	1	9	—	—
Millender	2,105	—	—	1	—	—	—
Beckenbaugh	532	26	—	1	11	—	38
Mannerfeldt	144	2.7	—	1		35	40
Urbaniak	93	—	—	—	—	—	20–90
Haber	116	1	—	1	10.3	34	51
Madden	250	(HP)[a] 1 (Orig)[b] 37	—	—	—	43	57
Blair, Shurr & Buckwalter	160	23	—	2	43	26.5	41.5

[a]HP = High Performance
[b]Orig = Original

ical studies. These issues include expectations of function, fracture rates, recurrent deformity, range of motion, and patient acceptance. The reader is advised that all studies do not report the same components of results or do not report results with consistency, leaving a void, as evidenced by Table 6-3.

Function

The issue of function is addressed in many different ways. Usually objective strength measurements are reported and function is inferred from a combination of range of motion, strength, and tasks usually described rather than observed. Since no clear-cut agreement exists as to evaluation of function, authors report results which are difficult to compare. Table 6.3 reports the work of 10 groups following spacer implants. Note the variability and absence in many columns, indicating the absence of information in many studies. Numbers of joints vary from 80 by Braun to more than 3,400 reported by Swanson.

Prosthetic Fracture

The data relative to prosthetic fracture are difficult to interpret. Criteria for fracture determination, as well as postoperative follow-up, make this reporting inconsistent. Changes in materials and design that occurred about 1974 further confuse the issue. Some authors believe that once the encapsulation process is complete, a fracture of the implant is really of little clinical consequence. Percentages of fracture reported vary from 0.9 percent by Swanson in 3,409 units to 37 percent by Madden and 26 percent by Beckenbaugh.

Infection

Infection following implant arthroplasty is very low no matter which study is cited. All but Blair[27] et al. report under 1 percent.

Recurrent Ulnar Deviation does occur and was reported to occur at a rate from 0 percent to 43 percent, depending on the author. Some authors believe that improper follow-up care and splinting, coupled with soft tissue imbalance and a progressive disease are responsible. No study clearly identified which of these proposed causes is more important.

Range of Motion

An improved range of motion is thought to be a universal outcome of implant arthroplasty. Nevertheless, some authors failed to report even postoperative range of motion. Preoperative range of motion is often unavailable, and therefore is not reported. Average reported preoperative range of motion ranged from 26.5 to 43°. Mention needs to be made concerning the concept of "active" versus "passive" range of motion when considering clinical results. Swanson used a passive technique, defined as "a force of 0.45 kg applied to the distal arm of the goniometer (10 cm from the axis of rotation) in the direction of flexion or extension, as the case may be." Other researchers[29] have used active motion, presumably without a passive assist, to define their range of motion.

Postoperative range of motion reported varies from 20° by Urbaniak to 70° by Braun. Reports of 40 to 55° average per joint are not uncommon. These results usually indicate that the change, although not large in degrees, occurs in the extension quadrant, as described by Mannerfeldt. These changes make the fingers useful to the patient, as they are able to open their hands to near MCP joint extension.

Patient Satisfaction

Subjective indices indicate that patient satisfaction following this procedure is quite high. Blair, Shurr, and Buckwalter reported 83 percent pain relief, 77 percent perceived increase in hand function, and 83 percent satisfaction with postoperative cosmesis. Given the variations in the presentation of clinical results, objective numbers are difficult to evaluate.

THE FUTURE

Newer designs and materials, like the pyrolitic carbons, ceramics, and ingrowth materials, will no doubt change future implants. More prospective controlled studies must be done to assess the role of the component parts in care of the rheumatoid hand, in order to better understand the relative importance of each. The contribution of the postoperative care specifically needs to be quantified and recorded. A sound test of function would allow a comparison of group to group, device to device, and outcome to outcome.

Knowledge of the benefits and limitations of the implant arthroplasty will permit both patient and team to approach the procedure with realistic expectations.

CASE STUDY

Molly S., a 58-year-old white female, has had rheumatoid arthritis for 15 years. She currently is in remission, has very little pain, and presents with a history of a steady decline in functional abilities bilaterally. Although she is right hand dominant, she reports doing most self-care tasks with her left hand.

M. S. has been followed by a rheumatologist and was last given gold 5 years ago. Her current medication is aspirin, 10 five-grain tablets per day. She is an unemployed home worker who walks unaided. M. S. is seeking consultation for answers to her questions about the possibility of implant surgery for the MCP joints. She states that in the last year her deformities have worsened to the point where she is unable to use her right hand to help herself in her home and wishes something to be done surgically to correct this situation.

Physical examination reveals severe destruction of her MCP joints, the right worse than the left. The joints of her right hand are totally dislocated volarly, with severe ulnar drift of all digits. She has 10° of active motion at the MCP joints, from 80° to 90°. Her ulnar deviation measures 30° and the proximal phalanges are slightly supinated. She has difficulty getting her ring and small fingers out of her palm; thus, holding objects on the power side of the hand difficult. Her proximal interphalangeal joints are much less involved, with 90° of active motion possible. She exhibits slight intrinsic tightness, probably due to the dislocation at the MCP joint. Her thumb has a mild zig-zag deformity, and x-ray reveals a slightly radially deviated wrist. She has severe synovial thickening over the MCP joints of the fingers and wrist, but all flexor and extensor tendons are intact and working. Sensation is within normal limits, and forearm pronation and supination measure 80° each.

M.S. was operated upon; silastic spacers were placed in the MCP joints of her right digits 2 to 5. In addition, a recentralization of the extensor tendons was accomplished. The abductor digiti minimi was sectioned at its musculocutaneous junction. A large bulky dressing was applied postoperatively and the hand and arm elevated for 4 days. Following removal of the bulky dressing, M.S. was fitted with a dorsal splint with extension outrigger and discharged to outpatient status. The splint maintained the fingers in −10° of MCP extension and slight radial deviation. Attention to a neutral position avoided any supination or pronation at the MCP joint. Early active motion exercises began to identify the flexors and extensors. Extensor exercise was completed using the intrinsic-minus maneuver, extending the MCP joint while holding the PIP joint flexed. Extreme care was taken not to allow the digits to deviate during flexion or extension. The patient was instructed in a basic postoperative care plan and instructed not to remove the splint for any reason.

The patient was seen three times a week during the first postoperative week. The splint was removed, the wound and splint were inspected and cleaned, and passive exercises were taught and supervised. By the end of the first week, the active motion at the MCP joints was only about 20°, although passive motion was 30°. A decision was made to implement flexion bands in an attempt to increase passive MCP flexion, and therefore the active MCP joint motion. The bands were introduced for 30 minutes initially, increasing to longer periods during the waking hours.

Weeks two and three involved visits three times per week. During these visits attention was focused on increasing flexion, as active extension continued to −5°. Passive stretching following heat application emphasized flexion. During active flexion exercises, splints kept the PIP joints from flexion, thus applying all effort to the MCP joint. By the end of the third week post-op, passive flexion of 65° was possible, with active flexion nearly 50° in all digits.

On post-op week four, M.S. was seen once a week. At the fourth week visit M.S. learned how to put on and take off the splint, how to align the flexion and extension outriggers, and what activities to avoid. In addition, passive exercise procedures were taught and witnessed, so she could exercise at home. Much time and effort was spent educating her as to the value of maintaining MCP alignment. Examples of relatively heavy activities assisted in giving the patient some functional perspective as to tasks to avoid yet at four weeks.

At 5 weeks M.S. lost 10° of flexion in the small finger MCP joint, from 50° to 40°. At that point, a stronger dynamic flexion cuff was initiated, progressing to overnight use. The program for the other digits remained the same, yielding 70° of passive flexion and about 50° of active MCP joint flexion. Active extension measured −7°, with good alignment and no rotation.

Daytime splinting was discontinued at week six. The therapist recommended that passive isolated exercise for the small finger MCP be done hourly. Night flexion bands were continued through week six, as a decision was made to emphasize flexion, in view of only 50° of active motion. M.S. was instructed to limit her activities to light work and to continue to avoid situations encouraging ulnar deviation of the MCP joints.

At 8 weeks, measurement revealed a relatively static situation of 50° of active flexion, from −20° to −70°. Alignment in radial-ulnar deviation and rotation was unchanged. M.S. was encouraged to resume her normal lifestyle and to use the hand as she needed to.

Follow-up continued at 6-month intervals through 2 years.

REFERENCES

1. Brannon EW, Kline G: Experiences with a finger-joint prosthesis. J Bone Joint Surg (Am) 41:87, 1959
2. Swanson AB, DeGroot Swanson G, Leonard J: Post-operative rehabilitation program in flexible implant arthroplasty of the digits. In Hunter JM, Schneider LH, Mackin EJ, Bell JA (eds): Rehabilitation of the Hand. CV Mosby Co, St Louis, 1978
3. Madden JW, DeVore G, Arem AJ: A rational post-operative management program for metacarpophalangeal joint implant arthroplasty. J Hand Surg 2:358, 1977
4. Flatt AE: Restoration of rheumatoid finger joint function, follow-up notes on articles previously published. J Bone Joint Surg (Am) 45:1101, 1963
5. Beckenbaugh, RD: Review and analysis of silicone-rubber metacarpophalangeal implants. J Bone Joint Surg (Am) 58:483, 1976
6. Swanson AB: Finger joint replacement by silicone rubber implants and the concept of implant fixation by encapsulation. Ann Rheum Dis 28: suppl. 47, 1969
7. Ashworth CR: Silicone-rubber interposition arthroplasty of the carpometacarpal joint of the thumb. J Hand Surg 2:345, 1977
8. Poppen NK: "Tie-in" trapezium prosthesis: long-term results. J Hand Surg 3:445, 1978
8a. Swanson AB: Disability arthritis at the base of the thumb. J Bone Joint Surg (Am) 54:3; 456, 1972

8b. Kessler I: Arthroplasty of the first carpometacarpal joint with a silicone implant. Plast Reconstr Surg 47:252, 1971

9. Ferlic DC: Degenerative arthritis of the carpometacarpal joint of the thumb: A clinical follow-up of eleven Niebauer prostheses. J Hand Surg 2:212, 1977

10. Burman MS: Vitallium cap arthroplasty of metacarpophalangeal and interphalangeal joints of fingers. Bull Hosp J Dis 1, 79:194

11. Flatt AE, Ellison MR: Restoration of rheumatoid finger joint function, III. J Bone Joint Surg (Am) 54:1317, 1972

12. Dryer RF: Proximal interphalangeal joint arthroplasty. In press

13. Blair EF, Shurr DG, Buckwalter JA: Metacarpophalangeal joint arthroplasty with a metallic hinged prosthesis. Clin Orthop 184:156, 1984

14. Girzadas DV, Clayton ML: Limitations of the use of metallic prosthesis in the rheumatoid hand. Clin Orthop 67:127, 1969

15. Swanson AB: Flexible implant arthroplasty for arthritis finger joints: rationale, technique, and results of treatment. J Bone Joint Surg (Am) 54:435, 1972

16. Mannerfelt L, Andersson K: Silastic arthroplasty of the metacarpophalangeal joints in rheumatoid arthritis. J Bone Joint Surg (Am) 57:484, 1975

17. Walker PS, Erhman MJ: Laboratory evaluation of a metal-plastic type of metacarpophalangeal joint prosthesis. Clin Orthop 112:349, 1975

18. Youm Y: Comparative study between normal metacarpophalangeal joint and prosthesis, I, kinematics of normal metacarpophalangeal joints. Proc 4th New England Bioengineering Conf, Yale University, New Haven, 1976

19. Gillespie TE: Biomechanical evaluation of metacarpophalangeal joint prosthesis designs. J Hand Surg 4:508, 1979

20. Flatt AE, The Care of the Rheumatoid Hand. CV Mosby Co, St Louis, 1963

21. Niebauer JJ, Landry RM: Dacron-silicone prosthesis for the metacarpalphalangeal and interphalangeal joints. Hand 3:55, 1971

22. Urbaniak JR: Prosthetic arthroplasty of the hand. Clin Orthop 104:9, 1974

23. Swanson AB: Implant resection arthroplasty of the proximal interphalangeal joint. Orthop Clin North Am 4:1007, 1970.

24. Reis ND, Calnan JS: Integral hinge joint. Ann Rheum Dis 28, (suppl.) 59, 1969

25. Strickland JW et al: Post-traumatic arthritis of the proximal interphalangeal joint. Ortho Rev 11:75, 1982

26. Dryer RD, Blair WF, Shuff DG, Buckwalter JA: Proximal interphalangeal joint arthroplasty. In press

27. Linscheid RL: Proximal interphalangeal joint arthroplasty. Mayo Clin Proc 54:227, 1979

28. Blair EF, Shuff DG, Buckwalter JA: Metacarpophalangeal joint implant with a silastic spacer. J Bone Joint Surg, 66-A: No. 3; 365, 1984

29. Fess EE, Harmon KS, Strickland JW, Steichen JB: Evaluation of the hand by objective measurement. In: Rehabilitation of the Hand, CV Mosby Co, St Louis, 1978

7 | Physical Capacity Evaluation and Work Therapy for Industrial Hand Injuries

Patricia L. Baxter

It has been estimated that every year, 100,000 industrial workers are permanently injured and more than 2 million miss one or more days of work because of job-related injuries or diseases. Each year 10 million workers require medical treatment or are forced into restricted activities because of such injuries. In 1980, approximately 400,000 work-related injuries were classified as hand and finger injuries.[1]

Industrial workers who sustain injuries at work appear to require longer periods of recovery than do patients who do not receive workman's compensation during their recovery stage. Many believe that the financial reimbursement for work-related accidents inhibits recovery in some patients. In a study on the variables influencing the hand injured worker's return to work, it was found that the patient receiving workman's compensation returned to work at a significantly lower rate than did patients who did not receive workman's compensation. In addition, many other variables such as occupational development, family history, and educational level were cited as significant factors influencing the patient's return to work. It was noted that referral of patients to occupational therapy had a positive effect on patients return to work.[2]

In 1982, a retrospective study was done on patients in the therapy program at the Hand Rehabilitation Center in Philadelphia. The length of time from injury to return to work was calculated for each patient and compared to the length of time from his initiation in the work tolerance program to his return to work. It was found that the length of time from injury to return to work was 63 percent longer for patients who received workman's compensation, as compared to privately funded patients. However, the most significant finding of the study was that the length of time in therapy for each group of patients and the rate of return to work for each group were not significantly different. The average length of therapy required for both patient groups was 6 weeks. Approximately 70 percent of the hand injured patients, on either workman's compensation coverage or private coverage, returned to work.[3]

HISTORY OF HAND THERAPY

The specialized concept of hand rehabilitation started during World War II. Military corps realized that patients with severe hand injury or a poor response to injury could benefit by the aggregation of such patients in a controlled environment where education, exercise, and functional activities could be encouraged by the therapist and other patients with hand problems.[4]

Therapeutic techniques used for rehabilitation of the hand-injured worker were further advanced by a hand surgeon in India. Paul Brand, MD, initiated the concept of comprehensive hand rehabilitation when he offered not only surgery but physical and occupational therapy to patients with Hansen's disease in India. Today, Dr. Brand's ideas have been incorporated into the comprehensive care offered at hand rehabilitation centers. The main goal of the surgeon and the therapist working in hand rehabilitation centers is to help the patient with an upper extremity injury to return to his former lifestyle, which includes work activities.

The services of hand rehabilitation teams include surgery and hand therapy. Great advances have been made in the past decade in the area of microvascular surgery, and this has affected a dramatic improvement in hand surgery techniques. Hand therapy techniques have advanced as well. Hand therapy provides primary care, work therapy, and specialized evaluations.

Primary care services include wound care and exercise, use of modalities and splints, and prosthetic fabrication.[5] For some patients primary care may be sufficient, and they may return to work after a brief postoperative phase of rehabilitation management. This chapter describes the services necessary for the majority of industrial workers treated at the Hand Rehabilitation Center in Philadelphia. These patients receive both primary care and work therapy to enable them to perform the heavy resistive work involved in manual labor and skilled labor.

Work therapy includes therapeutic activities, therapeutic exercise, and job simulation.[6] In work therapy, the patient performs progressive resistive work until he can perform job simulation adequately. At that time, he is evaluated for hand function ability, performance of job simulation tasks, and ability to perform the demands of work. This evaluation, called a physical capacity evaluation, is presented to the doctor so that upon discharge concrete recommendations can be provided to the patient's employer and insurance carrier concerning the patient's ability to perform his work.

WORK THERAPY

Therapeutic activities are used to improve the patient's range of motion and to initiate strengthening. Initially, therapeutic activities are light in resistance. Light hand activities may be chosen, using materials such as macrame or ceramic hand molding clay, to decrease swelling and improve tendon and muscle excursion. Strengthening occurs as the patient performs woodworking. The prolonged grasp of the woodworking handle is an exercise which is safely initiated for beginning more resistive exercises. Woodworking is used to improve endurance.

Therapeutic exercises also involve the patient in resistive work to improve strength and endurance. The patient may perform weight lifting, pulley exercises, or resistive hand exercises. A progressive resistive pulley exerciser, the Mini-gym*, is used to promote bilateral muscle conditioning. Hand exercises used to promote strengthening include weight well exercise and wrist exercises.[7] Putty and the hand helper are given to the patient to enable him to perform resistive hand exercises while at home.

Job simulation is carried out with the BTE Work Simulator.† The BTE Work Simulator is a device that can be adjusted to simulate the specific motions required of the patient in his work.[8] It has a variable resistance mechanism that can be adjusted so that the patient is required to work against a specific force in order to move the tool attachment on the machine. There are 16 tool attachments that can be used to simulate the various job requirements of each patient.

SPECIALIZED EVALUATIONS

Specialized evaluations are necessary to evaluate the patient's ability to function at home and at work. Specialized evaluations include sensibility evaluations, electromyographic studies, and nerve velocity conduction studies, evaluation of daily living skills, and physical capacity evaluation.[9] The physical capacity evaluation, as described in this article, is provided by the work therapy section of the hand therapy department.

Physical Capacity Evaluation

The physical capacity evaluation documents the patient's objective hand function, such as strength and range of motion. The patient's physical abilities and limitations are further described through the use of standardized tests. During the physical capacity evaluation, the patient is observed performing job requirements. Based on the objective findings from the standardized tests, the hand measurements, and subjective observation of the patient's performance of job tasks, the therapist reports the patient's ability to return to work to the surgeon. The surgeon makes the final determination as to the patient's ability to physically perform his job adequately.

The physical capacity evaluation has three basic components. The hand function evaluation is the first component. The therapist evaluates the patient's range of motion, grip and pinch strength, and sensibility.

The second component is administration of standardized tests. There are several standardized tests available. The following tests are used regularly at the Hand Rehabilitation Center in Philadelphia: the Valpar Upper Extremity Range-of-Motion Work Sample, the Valpar Simulated Assembly Work Sample, the Valpar Small Tools Me-

---

*Mini-gym, Inc, 901 West Lexinton, Box 266, Independence, MO 64051.
†Baltimore Therapeutic Equipment Co, 1201 Bernard Drive, Baltimore, MD 21223

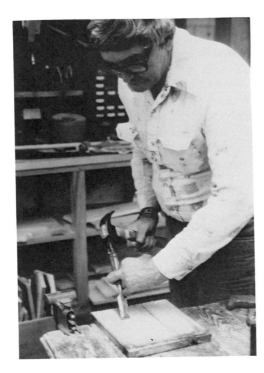

Fig. 7-1. A stable grasp of tools achieved with the patient's injured hand.

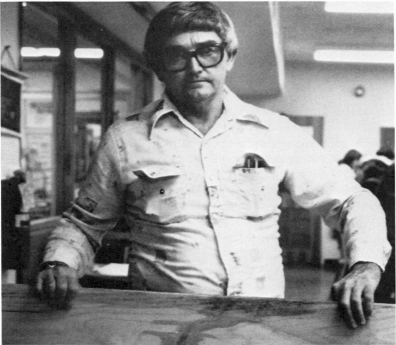

Fig. 7-2.   The patient could lift and carry the amount of lumber required at his job.

chanical Work Sample, the Purdue Pegboard, and the Minnesota Rate of Manipulation Test.[10]

The third component is the most important. This section requires the therapist to observe the patient performing the physical demands of his job. Physical tasks can be broken down into physical motions and simulation of physical activities. The *Dictionary of Occupational Titles* is a reference the therapist can utilize to obtain information on the physical demands of each patient's job.[11]

The patient is observed in this section of the evaluation while he lifts weighted boxes and carries them a distance of 25 ft. He begins by lifting 5 lb and progresses to the maximum weight he can safely lift. The patient performs the tasks with his uninvolved hand first and then with his injured hand. Bilateral lifting is required as well. If the patient's job requires repetitive lifting, the patient is observed as he performs repetitive lifting throughout the evaluation time period. Other physical tasks the patient is observed performing depend on his job requirements. Physical demands include standing, sitting, walking, climbing, bending, stooping, reaching, handling, and manipulating.

The Work Simulator is also used in this evaluation of the patient's ability to perform his work. This instrument is designed to quantitatively assess the patient's work output and power output as he performs job simulation.

The patient is required to perform job simulation with his dominant hand and his non-dominant hand for extended periods of time until he becomes fatigued. The Work Simulator calculates the amount of work output by multiplying the force the patient exerts by the distance he rotates the tool attachment on the machine. Power output is calculated by dividing the time the patient works into the force multiplied by the distance. Recommendations concerning the patient's ability to perform his job are based on the ease of performance and the demonstrated endurance.

CASE STUDIES

Several case examples will be presented to illustrate the appropriate application of work therapy techniques and the recommendations determined from the patient's participation in a physical capacity evaluation.

Case 1

The first case is a 38-year-old right-handed carpenter. His left hand went into a power saw, amputating his left thumb and severely lacerating his left palm. He had initial skin grafting to the palm, but painful neuromas developed. He had further surgical procedures which included resection of the neuromas, repair of the radial digital nerve to the index finger, split-thickness skin grafts to the left palm, and deepening of the first web space. The patient demonstrated full range of motion of his digits after he participated in a comprehensive hand rehabilitation program, which included primary care and work therapy.

During the physical capacity evaluation, coordination ability of the patient was evaluated with one of the Valpar Work Samples. The patient was observed to

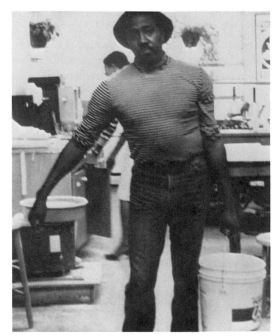

Fig. 7-3. At work, the patient had to lift and carry a heavy bucket filled with material liquid.

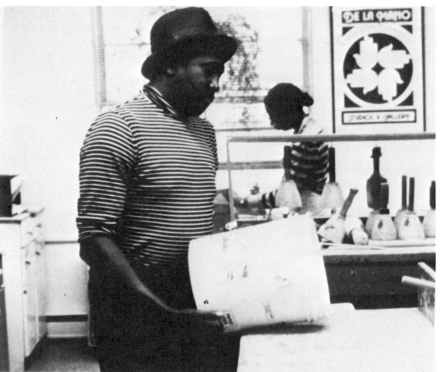

Fig. 7-4. Next, he had to pour the material into the machine.

compensate for the lack of an opposable thumb by opposing with his index finger to his middle finger. He demonstrated adequate ability to handle the tools of his trade, carpentry (Fig. 7-1), and he was able to lift and carry lumber of the same weight as required at work (Fig. 7-2). Therefore, it was recommended that he return to his regular job. He has been working successfully for several months at his regular job. He is scheduled to return to the Hand Rehabilitation Center for follow-up evaluation in 1 year.

Case 2

The next patient is a 39-year-old machine operator who sustained multiple amputations of his right digits. The patient's hand was crushed between two rollers of a machine that fabricated metal parts. The patient's index, middle, and ring fingers were amputated proximal to his proximal interphalangeal joints. There was a nail avulsion of the fifth finger. The patient's thumb was not injured. Metacarpophalangeal joint capsulotomies were performed to improve the patient's flexion.

The patient demonstrated 30 lb of grip strength with his right injured hand as compared to 120 lb with his left hand.

He participated in primary care as well as a work therapy program. In the work therapy program he used the Work Simulator to regain strength and endurance. During the physical capacity evaluation, the patient's job duties were identified. Job duties included lifting and carrying a 32 lb bucket with his uninjured hand (Fig. 7-3). Then he had to pour the material from the bucket into the machine rollers using both hands (Fig. 7-4). He used a rod to spread this material evenly onto the rollers. The patient's job was simulated by using common available objects. It was recommended that the patient return to his regular job, which he has done successfully.

Case 3

The next case is a 48-year-old janitor who sustained a crush injury to his right hand when his hand was caught in the rollers of a machine. He had amputations of his fourth and fifth digits and a partial amputation of his middle finger (Fig. 7-5 A,B). Fusion of the index and middle finger metacarpophalangeal joints were necessary due to unstable fractures. However, the fusions were not sufficient to support comfortably the lifting requirements of his job (Fig. 7-6). Therefore, a protective splint was designed for the patient to use during strenuous work (Fig. 7-7). He was referred to a prosthetist for a permanent prosthesis and then was able to return to work.

SUMMARY

In summary, the physical capacity evaluation is utilized to assess the patient's ability to return to work, through administration of hand function tasks, standardized

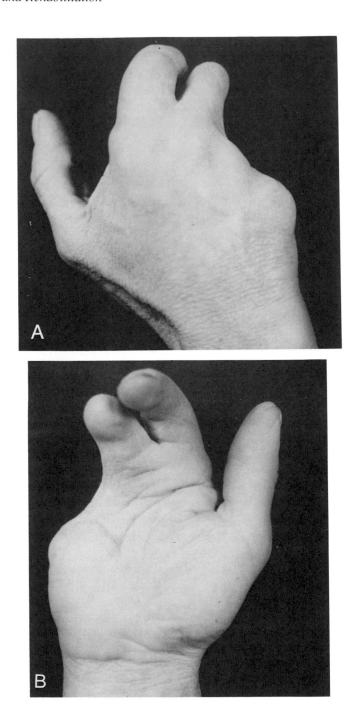

Fig. 7-5. (A) The patient's right hand was crushed in a machine resulting in partial and complete amputation of the digits. (B) Fusion of multiple joints was necessary.

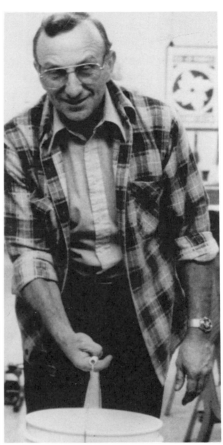

Fig. 7-6. The patient could not use his right hand to lift heavy objects at work.

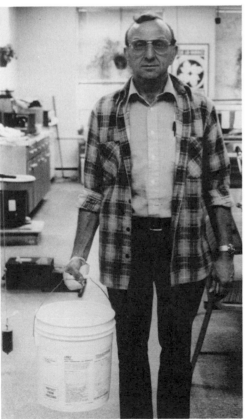

Fig. 7-7. Unilateral and bilateral lifting was possible with the right hand when the patient wore the splint.

tests, and observation of the patient performing his job requirements. This evaluation is usually performed after the patient has participated in a comprehensive hand rehabilitation program, including primary care and work therapy. The recommendations vary according to the patient's performance on the evaluation. The therapist may recommend that the patient return to his former job or to a modified job. Other recommendations may include the use of adaptive equipment to enable the patient to perform his job duties, or the need for further surgery or therapy may be indicated through the patient's performance.

REFERENCES

1. Sloane L: What is workmen's compensation? Am J Nurs 78:957, 1978.
2. Bear-Lehman J: Factors affecting return to work after hand injury. Am J Occup Ther 37:189, 1983
3. Baxter PL, Ballard M, Fried S: A multi-perspective profile of patients involved in a work tolerance program. Unpublished Paper, Philadelphia, 1982
4. Lankford L, Carter PR, Magnenat GF: The value of a hand therapy unit in rehabilitating the disabled hand. Unpublished Paper, Dallas, 1977
5. McEntee P et al: The hand rehabilitation center in Philadelphia, a private comprehensive program. p. 939. In Hunter JM et al (eds): Rehabilitation of the Hand. 2nd Ed. CV Mosby Co, St Louis, 1983
6. Baxter PL, McEntee P: The physical capacity evaluation. p. 909. In Hunter JM et al (eds): Rehabilitation of the Hand. 2nd Ed. CV Mosby Co, St Louis, 1983
7. Hunter JM: Dedication. p. x. In Hunter JM et al (eds): Rehabilitation of the Hand. CV Mosby Co, St Louis, 1978
8. Curtis RM, Engalitcheff J: A work simulator for rehabilitating the upper extremity—preliminary report. J Hand Surg 6:499, 1981
9. Baxter PL, Fried S: The work tolerance program of the hand rehabilitation center. p. 889. In Hunter JM et al (eds): Rehabilitation of the Hand. 2nd Ed. CV Mosby Co, St Louis, 1983
10. Baxter PL, Ballard M: Evaluation of the hand by functional tests. p. 91. In Hunter JM et al (eds): Rehabilitation of the Hand. 2nd Ed. CV Mosby Co, St Louis, 1983
11. US Department of Labor Dictionary of Occupational Titles, 3rd Ed., Vol. I and II. Washington, DC, 1968

8 | The Painful Hand

Valerie Holdeman Lee

Many patients with devastating injuries to the upper extremity do not experience pain to a degree that interferes significantly with rehabilitation. Yet others with seemingly minor injuries develop disabling pain that progresses from acute to chronic. The goal of hand rehabilitation is to restore motion and function in an orderly fashion. The hand therapist must have an awareness of what is an appropriate amount of discomfort following an injury, versus disproportionate pain that has a potential for becoming either a chronic pain problem or for developing into a reflex sympathetic dystrophy.

Classically, acute pain is defined as pain of less than 3 to 6 months duration, while chronic pain persists beyond that amount of time. Acute pain might also be defined as pain that is normally expected following an injury and serves a function by giving feedback to therapist and patient to prevent further damage to healing tissue. Chronic pain, on the other hand, does not serve a purpose, lasts longer than is expected, and precipitates a continued disability, both physical and psychological, to the patient.

PAIN TRANSMISSION THEORIES

Over the last decade a great deal of research has been carried out concerning the mechanism of pain transmission. A major theory was proposed by Melzack and Wall in 1965.[1] They postulated that the perception of pain is dependent upon the balance of small nociceptive fibers (A delta and C fibers) and large myelinated fibers (A alpha and beta fibers) in the substantia gelatinosa (laminae II and III) of the dorsal horn. Increased activity of the large afferent fibers closes the gate and prevents the transmission of pain through presynaptic inhibition of the nocioceptive fibers. Higher brain functions are also capable of affecting the perception of pain.[2,3]

While controversy exists concerning the complete validity of the gate control theory, it continues to serve as a working model of pain transmission and is proposed as a rationale for many modalities used in pain management, such as conventional TENS, massage, and application of heat.[4]

147

ENDOGENOUS OPIATES

In 1971 Avram Goldstein developed a method for the detection of highly specific opiate receptors in neuronal membranes and in the mouse brain.[5] In 1975 opiate-like substances termed endorphins (endogenous morphine) were discovered in the brain.[6] Both acupuncture-like TENS and acupuncture are believed to relieve pain through the release of endorphins. Naloxone, a morphine antagonist, reverses pain relief achieved through acupuncture and low-frequency (acupuncture-like) TENS, while it does not reverse pain relief achieved through conventional TENS or hypnosis.

More recently, the use of cold laser for pain relief has been based on the release of endorphins.[8] While this modality may hold promise, more research in its use and effectiveness is necessary.

It should also be noted that naloxone reverses the placebo effect, indicating that endorphins are brought into play by other than physical means of stimulation.[6,9]

PSYCHOLOGICAL ASPECTS OF PAIN PERCEPTION

The psychological impact of a hand injury can be severe. The hand has often been referred to as a highly emotionally charged body part. Frequently the patient first sees his or her injured hand in therapy, devoid of bandage or surgical dressings. The patient is not always prepared, and many patients become nauseous and light headed. The therapist must anticipate these problems and be supportive.

Anxiety and fear play an important part in the perception of pain.[3] By relieving anxiety, pain can be reduced. Patient education concerning the injury, subsequent surgery, and rehabilitation can relieve part of this fear. Experiments have also shown that anxiety can be reduced by granting the patient a certain degree of control. For instance, when the therapist asks for an active motion, the patient is in control. Also, when performing passive motion, ask the patient to give you feedback as to the amount of pain or discomfort experienced. Always maintain eye contact with your patients.

Other factors such as previous experiences, pending litigation, hostility towards the employer, and the patient's culture affect the perception of pain. It is the high degree of subjectivity that makes pain so difficult to assess and treat effectively.

THE GROUP SETTING

Hand therapy lends itself well to a group setting. New patients with a severe injury, when introduced to other hand injured patients, almost universally express amazement at the number of people in a similar situation. By communicating with others in different states of rehabilitation, the patient feels less alone and more optimistic about the future (Fig. 8-1).

The therapist is, of course, an integral part of this group. He or she must be supportive but not overly sympathetic. Behavior modification should be an integral part of treatment. Perhaps oversimplified, the therapist responds to positive behavior and gives no response to negative behavior.

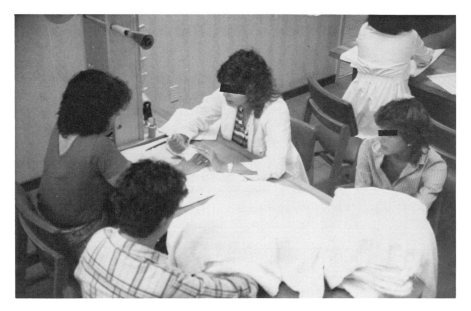

Fig. 8-1. Treatment of the pain patient in a group setting facilitates a positive attitude toward recovery.

In order to achieve best results from the use of a group setting and behavior modification, careful scheduling of patients is essential. Patients who would have a negative effect on others in the group are first treated alone or with only very positive patients, until they can be integrated into the group.

Group therapy has another benefit: By listening to each patient communicating with others, the therapist receives a great deal of information about the patient's attitudes toward injury, pain, employer, vocation, and the physician. The intuitive therapist then has a better insight into the patient, and should be better equipped to offer appropriate treatment.

THE ACUTELY INJURED HAND

Pain management begins in the emergency room, where medical treatment is first received—either through the use of analgesics or peripheral nerve block. The hand surgeon then attempts to minimize postoperative pain and edema through careful handling of tissue and control of intraoperative bleeding. Following surgery, the hand is placed in a compressive bandage and elevated.

Edema is the body's first response to injury, and while the early stages of edema are reversible, the resulting fibrosis is not. This hypomobility results in decreased sensory input of large afferent fibers, "opens the gate," and results in increased pain.

Patients must be encouraged to elevate their hands above the heart as frequently as possible. Propping the hand on pillows at night helps to prevent dependency.

Active motion, retrograde massage, and the use of ice aid in reduction of edema. The effectiveness of edema control is best monitored with the use of the volumeter.

Thermoelastic, Isotoner,* and surgical gloves may also be used to assist in edema reduction.[10]

PAIN CONTROL FOR EARLY MOBILIZATION

The timing of immobilization/mobilization is determined by the injury or surgical procedure. However, the *rate* of rehabilitation is often affected by the degree of pain perceived by the patient, as continued mobilization or lack of adequate mobilization past an optimum time decreases the chances of achieving the desired result; pain control is a critical factor in rehabilitation.

CAPSULOTOMIES—TENOLYSIS

Following tenolysis and capsulotomies, early motion is essential to promote optimum tendon glide and maximal joint motion. Active motion usually begins within 24 hours and is understandably associated with acute pain, secondary to the surgical procedure.

In the first 24 to 72 hours cold may be applied in the form of cold packs in elevation to decrease capillary permeability, thereby slowing fluid leakage from ruptured vessels and preventing an increase in edema. The TENS may also be used if active motion is being hampered by the patient's pain. As it is necessary for the patient to exercise several times daily, it may be beneficial to have the patient rent the TENS unit for home use.

Another method used for pain relief in facilitating active motion in patients following tenolysis or capsulotomy is described by Schneider and Mackin.[12] This method employs an indwelling polyethylene catheter that is left in the area of tenolysis at the time of surgery. Small amounts of local anesthetic are instilled into the operated area to decrease discomfort when exercising.[11]

Care must be taken when treating patients following tenolysis and/or capsulotomy. During tenolysis the vascular supply to the tendon may be disturbed, leaving the tendon in a weakened condition. Over-zealous treatment may result in a ruptured tendon. Overly aggressive therapy following capsulotomy may result in increased edema, which will reduce range of motion. Close rapport with the surgeon and an understanding of the surgical procedure is mandatory.

Another hand injury that is mobilized early following surgery is primary repair of flexor tendons in Zone II. The digits are mobilized at 3 to 5 days according to a specific regime,[12] and the patient remains in a dorsal splint to prevent stretch or rupture of the repaired tendons. This immobilization precludes the use of ice to reduce edema; however, retrograde massage of the digits and elevation are useful. Tendon repairs without sensory nerve damage or extensive soft tissue damage should not result in a significant

---

*Aris Gloves, 417 5th Ave, New York, NY 10016

amount of pain. However, should the patient complain of burning pain or paresthesias in the thumb, index and middle finger, the degree of wrist flexion could be compressing the median nerve under the flexor retinaculum. In this instance, the physician should be notified immediately. Often by decreasing the degree of wrist flexion, the compression on the median nerve will be released sufficiently to eliminate paresthesias.

FRACTURES

Stable fractures of the metacarpals and phalanges are often mobilized at 5 days to 2 weeks. Early protected motion results in decreasing edema, increasing tendon excursion, and reducing the likelihood of extension contractures of the metacarpophalangeal joints and flexion contractures of the proximal interphalangeal joints.

Moist heat in the form of hot packs may be used with elevation to increase the extensibility of collagen when combined with mild stretching.[4] They should be given with the extremity in elevation and removed at 8 to 10 minutes for maximum benefit. It is postulated that the analgesic effect of heat is due to either a counterirritant effect or perhaps to the release of endorphins. Lehmann et al. measured the pain threshold before and after heat application. The pain threshold was found to be elevated after heating.

These patients may complain of a deep, diffuse aching pain, which is to be expected from the healing periosteum. The deep pain may produce reflex complications such as sweating, bradycardia, hypotension, and nausea.[13] Early protected motion is characterized by active motion while the therapist externally supports the fracture site.

Complaints by the patient of severe, sharp pain with active motion may indicate instability of the fracture, and the surgeon should be informed.

LACERATIONS AND REPAIR OF PERIPHERAL NERVES

Following repair of peripheral nerves, the hand is generally immobilized in a protective position for 3 weeks. Injury to strictly motor nerves is not painful, and repair of complete lacerations to a mixed nerve is not generally painful until the process of reinnervation begins. This pain is due to the presence of hypersensitive immature regenerating axons at the site of the lesion,[14] and will dissipate as the axons mature. It is referred to as *hypopathia*. Generally, the pain is not severe, and responds well to heat, massage, and desensitization techniques.[15]

PAINFUL NEUROMAS

Neuromas develop at the proximal stump of a severed sensory nerve. While neuroma formation is inevitable, not all neuromas are painful.

Painful neuromas contain inadequately sheathed and highly sensitive regenerating axons.[14] This absence of large fiber activity "opens the gate" and results in the percep-

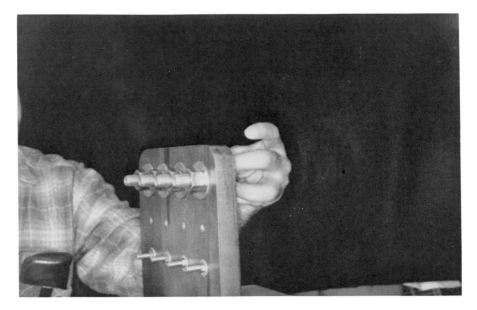

Fig. 8-2.   This patient displays an "extensor habitus" pattern as he attempts a functional activity.

tion of pain. The use of high rate-conventional TENS is beneficial and must be applied *proximal* to the neuroma along the nerve's pathway in order to recruit the large afferent fibers to close the gate.

There is also some clinical suggestion that ultrasound may reduce the sensitivity of a neuroma, although the exact mechanism is not known.

When neuromas occur in the volar surface of the distal phalanx, the patient will go to great lengths to avoid using the finger in a normal manner. This can lead to what is commonly termed "extensor habitus," particularly when the involved digit is the index finger (Fig. 8-2).

Desensitization techniques are again necessary and the patient may be encouraged to use his finger by protecting the sensitive area with a small splint of elastomer* and Coban† (Fig. 8-3). The deep pressure of the Coban is well tolerated, and the patient will then more willingly perform normal prehensile patterns.

Neuromas that are not only painful when touched but elicit pain with motion may be imbedded in scar. If TENS, desensitization, and tincture of time do not decrease sensitivity, the surgeon may elect to resect or transpose the neuroma to a better protected area.

CARPAL TUNNEL SYNDROME

Carpal tunnel syndrome is the result of pressure on the median nerve under the flexor retinaculum. This may result from increased volume in the carpal canal due to edema or tenosynovitis of the flexor tendons.

---

*WFR Corp, PO Box 215, Ramsey, NJ 07446
†3M Corp, Medical Products Division, St Paul, MN.

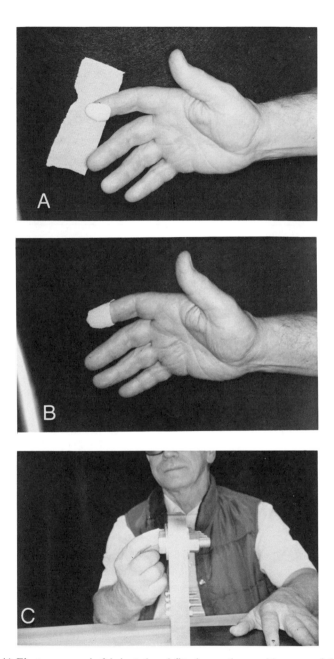

Fig. 8-3. (A) Elastomer cap is fabricated and fitted over the sensitive area of the index digit. (B) The elastomer cap is secured with Coban to permit full digit function. (C) With the elastomer cap in place, the patient is able to use the sensitive index tip in performing a functional activity.

The patient will complain of paresthesias generally in the thumb, index, and middle finger and in half of the ring finger. The pain will be described as burning in nature and will be worse at night, when driving, and when reading the newspaper. A positive Phalen's test is elicited when the wrist is flexed and when the patient reports increasing numbness. A "reverse Phalen's" test is positive when increasing numbness is reported when the wrist is maximally extended. A positive Phalen's results from increased pressure on the median nerve, while a positive reverse Phalen's results from traction the median nerve when the wrist is extended.

CTS is classically confirmed from nerve conduction studies and by a decrease in two-point discrimination. However, by using the Semmes-Weinstein monofilament,* compression on the median nerve can be discerned clinically.

When symptoms of compression occur acutely, the physician should be informed immediately so that measures can be taken to reduce the compression. Early reduction of symptoms by simple remedies such as loosening a cast can prevent an acute problem from becoming chronic. Compression of the median nerve is often a predisposing factor leading to a reflex sympathetic dystrophy.

Chronic CTS is often treated with TENS, ultrasound, phonophoresis, and night splinting in 10 to 15° of extension. Patients whose jobs require repetitive motion may need to change vocation or alter their pattern of motion.

Carpal tunnel syndrome may ultimately lead to release of the flexor retinaculum and/or neurolysis of the median nerve. The use of TENS and desensitization is often beneficial postoperatively.

De QUERVAINS' SYNDROME

De Quervain's syndrome is defined as stenosing tenosynovitis of the extensor pollicis brevis and the abductor pollicis longus in the first dorsal compartment. It occurs more often in women than in men and is often found in people whose jobs require repetitive stress.

Patients with De Quervains syndrome will exhibit a positive Finkelstein test. This test is performed by asking the patient to flex his adducted thumb maximally, then to flex the digits over the thumb and ulnarly deviate the wrist (Fig. 8-4). A positive Finkelstein occurs when the patient complains of severe pain over the second compartment.

Conservative treatment generally consists of a period of immobilization (the splint used must immobilize the wrist as well as the MP and IP joints) followed by gradual mobilization. Steroid injections and anti-inflammatory medication may also be indicated. Adjunctive modalities include ultrasound, heat, and ice massage. Ultrasound should be used under water to prevent periosteal burning due to lack of subcutaneous tissue.

The TENS is particularly beneficial if there is evidence of involvement of the dorsal branch of the superficial radial nerve, which is a potentially dangerous condition and can lead to a reflex sympathetic dystrophy.

---

*Research Designs, Inc., 9811 Harwin Dr, Houston, Texas 77036

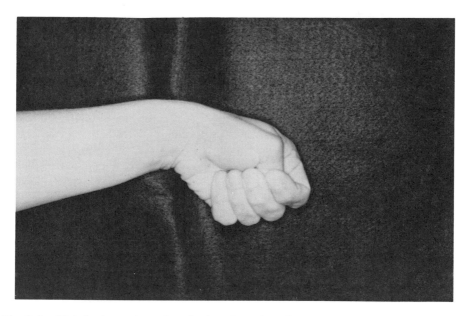

Fig. 8-4. Finkelstein test is perfomed when the patient displays symptoms of stenosing teno-synovitis of the first dorsal compartment.

When conservative treatment fails, surgical release of the first compartment is indicated.

REFLEX SYMPATHETIC DYSTROPHY

In 1864 Weir Mitchell first described the severe pain following nerve injuries that occurred during the Civil War.[16] In 1867 Mitchell used the term "causalgia" from the Greek words for "burning pain."[17] In 1940 Homans used the term "minor causalgia" to describe the pain and trophic changes from non-nerve injuries.[18]

In 1977 Lankford and Thompson classified various clinical types of reflex sympathetic dystrophies.[19] Injury to a major mixed nerve was termed major causalgia and injury to a sensory nerve, minor causalgia. Injuries that did not specifically involve nerves were termed traumatic dystrophies, with minor and major referring to the severity of the trauma. Shoulder-hand syndrome was set apart as a separate entity in this classification.

Lankford also states three necessary factors which need to be present for RSD to occur: (1) a painful lesion, (2) diathesis, or susceptibility of the patient, and (3) an abnormal autonomic reflex.

While there exist an indefinite number of possibilities for a painful lesion, the most common causes in the upper extremity are: (1) crush injuries, (2) injuries to the median nerve at the wrist, (3) injuries to the superficial radial nerve, (4) lacerations or crush injuries to digital nerves, and (5) Colles' fracture.

The two most common elective procedures to be followed by RSD are decompression of the median nerve at the wrist and palmar fasciectomy for Dupuytren's contracture.

Lankford defined *diathesis* as a bodily condition, a systemic characteristic, an inherent tendency, or a constitutional predisposition. While certain personality types may demonstrate more of a tendency to develop RSD, the presence of chronic pain may also promote emotional change.[20,21]

It is the practice of some centers to screen pain patients by means of the Minnesota Multiphonic Personality Inventory; however, according to several studies, the MMPI cannot be used to differentiate between patients with organic and psychogenic pain.[22]

The third requirement of Lankford is the presence of an abnormal autonomic reflex. While a sympathetic reflex is a part of the initial response to injury, when the sympathetic reflex continues or is more pronounced than normal because of an abnormal feedback mechanism, an atypical sympathetic reflex ensues.[19]

While the exact mechanism determining the etiology of RSD is not known, certainly the most striking characteristic is pain that is disproportionate to the injury. The pain is most commonly described as burning in nature, which indicates C-fiber activity.[13,23] The pain often radiates proximally into the shoulder, axilla, and anterior chest wall. The majority of the patients exhibit some degree of cold intolerance.

The signs most commonly seen are edema, decreased joint motion, hyperesthesia, and changes in skin color or texture. Redness may be noted over the MP and IP joints.[13]

The use of stellate ganglion blocks and IV or intra-arterial reserpine have been reported to give the best results when used early[24,25] and on patients who have a vascular component to their pain. In later stages, when the pain is due to chronic compression of the nerve, the patients do not respond well to either.

Promising results using implanted electrodes on peripheral nerves have been reported in the literature,[25,26] when use of the TENS brought only partial relief.

CLINICAL TREATMENT

A case report on a child with RSD was reported recently.[27] The patient developed a RSD after striking her elbow on a chair and was treated with low frequency TENS at acupuncture and auriculotherapy points with excellent results. Melzack achieved similar results with brief intense electrical stimulation delivered to acupuncture points.[28] Perhaps the most important factor in treating patients with RSD or potential RSD is early recognition and aggressive treatment.

Alone or in conjunction with sympathetic blocks, reserpine, and anti-inflammatory medication, sensory bombardment to close the gate is essential. Massage, TENS, moist heat in elevation, gentle active exercises, and static and dynamic splinting must be incorporated into the rehabilitation program.

Static splints should be worn only at night, and dynamic splints must not increase pain or edema. Elevation and active use of the extremity is encouraged. Most importantly, there should be no painful manipulation of the hand by the therapist.

REFERENCES

1. Melzack R, Wall PD: Pain mechanisms: A new theory. Science 150:971, 1965
2. Melzack R: Myofascial trigger points: Relation to acupuncture and mechanisms of pain. Arch Phys Med Rehabil 62:114, March, 1981
3. Melzack R: The perception of pain. Sci Am 204(2):41, 1961
4. Lehman JF: Therapeutic Heat and Cold. 3rd Ed. Williams & Wilkins, Baltimore, 1982
5. Goldstein A: Opioid peptides (Endorphins) in pituitary and brain. Science 193:1081, Sept 17, 1976
6. Bishop B: Pain: Its physiology and rationale for management. Part II. Phys Ther 60(1):21, Jan. 1980
7. Abram SE, Reynolds AC, Cusick JF: Failure of naloxone to reverse analgesia from transcutaneous electrical stimulation in patients with chronic pain. Anesth Analg 60(2):81, Feb. 1981
8. Kleinkort J, Foley R: Laser: A Preliminary Report on Its Use in Physical Therapy, 1-19
9. Richards MD: Causalgia, a centennial review. Arch Neurol 16:339, April 1967
10. Hunter JM, Mackin EJ: Edema and bandaging. Hunter JM, Schneider L, Mackin E, and Bell J (eds) Rehabilitation of the Hand. p. 113. CV Mosby Co, St Louis, 1978
11. Shealy NC, Maurer D: Transcutaneous nerve stimulation for control of pain. Surg Neurol 2: 45, Jan. 1974
12. Schneider L, Mackin E: Tenolysis. p. 229. In Hunter JM, Schneider L, Mackin E, and Bell J (eds): Rehabilitation of the Hand. CV Mosby Co, St Louis, 1978
13. Reuler J, Girard, D, Nardone D: The chronic pain syndrome: Misconceptions and management," Ann Intern Med 93:588, 1980
14. Simons DG: Myofascial trigger points: A need for understanding. Arch Phys Med Rehabil 62:97, March 1981
15. Nashold BS, Maron C, Freedman H: Dorsal column stimulation for control of pain. J Neurosurg 36:590, May, 1972
16. Mitchell SW, Morehouse GR, Keen WW: Gunshot Wounds and Other Injuries of Nerves. JB Lippincott Co, Philadelphia, 1864
17. Rook J, Pesch RN, Keeler E: Chronic pain and the questionable use of the Minnesota Multiphasic Personality Inventory. Arch Phys Med Rehabil 62:373, August, 1981
18. Homans J: Minor causalgia: A hyperesthetic neurovascular syndrome. N Engl J Med 222 (21):870 May 23, 1940
19. Lankford L, Thompson E: Reflex Sympathetic Dystrophy, Upper and Lower Extremity: Diagnosis and Management, Orthopedic Complications. 168-178
20. Merskey H, Boyd D: Emotional adjustment and chronic pain. Pain 5:173, 1978
21. Sunderland S: Painful Sequelae of Injuries to Peripheral Nerves.
22. Russek AS, Mannheimer JS: How TENS works. Rx Home Care 22, Nov. 1982
23. Bishop B: Pain: Its physiology and rationale for management. Part I. Phys Ther 60 (1):13, Jan. 1980
24. Nashold BS, Goldner JL, Mullen JB, Bright DS: Long-term pain control by direct peripheral nerve stimulation. J Bone Joint Surg (Am) 64 (1):1, Jan. 1982
25. Omer GE, Thomas Lt Col S: The management of chronic pain syndromes in the upper extremity Clin Orthop 104:37, Oct. 1974
26. Law JD, Swett J, Kirsch W: Retrospective analysis of 22 patients with chronic pain treated by peripheral nerve stimulation. J Neurosurg 52:482, April 1980

27. Leo KC: Use of electrical stimulation at acupuncture points for the treatment of reflex sympathetic dystrophy in a child. A case report. Phys Ther 63 (6):957, June, 1983
28. Melzack R: Prolonged relief of pain by brief intense transcutaneous somatic stimulation. Pain 1: 357, 1975

SUGGESTED READING

Barnes R: The role of sympathectomy in the treatment of causalgia. J Bone Joint Surg 35B (2): 172, May 1855

Cheng RSS: Electroacupuncture On Cat Spinal Cord Neurons and Conscious Mice: A New Hypothesis. 1-17

Doleys DM, Crocker M, Patton D: Response of patients with chronic pain to exercise quotas. Phys Ther 62 (8):1111, Aug. 1982

Drucker WR, Hubay CA, Holden WD, Bukovnic JA: Pathogenesis of post traumatic sympathetic dystrophy. Am J Surg 97:454, April 1959

Erikkson M, Sjolund B: Acupuncturelike electroanalgesia in TNS-resistant chronic pain. p. 575. In Zolterman Y (ed): Sensory Functions of the Skin. 1976

Jeffcoate WJ: Brain peptides and pain sensation. Am Heart J 99 (1):1. CV Mosby Co, St Louis, January, 1980

Kleinert HE, Cole NM, Wayne L, Harvey R, Kutz J, Atasoy E: Post-traumatic sympathetic dystrophy. Orthop Clin North Am 4 (4):917. October, 1973

Liebeskind JC: Multiple mechanisms of pain inhibition intrinsic to the central nervous system. J Anesth 54 (6):445, June, 1981

Marx JL: Neurobiology: Researchers high on endogenous opiates. Science 193:1227, Sept 24, 1976

Melzack R, Guite S, Gonshor A: Relief of dental pain by ice massage of the hand. CMA Journal 122, 189, January 26, 1980

Roesch R, Ulrich D: Physical therapy management in the treatment of chronic pain. Phys Ther 60 (1):53. January, 1980

Sunderland S: Nerves and Nerve Injuries. Churchill Livingstone, London, 1968

Sweet WH, Wespic JG: Control of pain by local electrical stimulation for suppression. Ariz Med 26:1042, Dec. 1969

VanderArk GD, McGrath K: Transcutaneous electrical stimulation treatment of postoperative pain. Am J Surg 130:338, Sept 1975

9 | Splinting Principles For Hand Injuries

Maureen Gateley Gribben

The specialized area of hand splinting has traditionally been seen as the province of the occupational therapist, rather than as that of the physical therapist. The growth of the field of hand rehabilitation during the last decade and the establishment of the American Society of Hand Therapists in 1977 have both served to bring physical and occupational therapists together in pursuit of the common goal of the conservative management of upper extremity of dysfunction.

As practicing therapists, we see hand injury and pathology in a variety of clinical settings. For this reason, a knowledge of hand anatomy and kinesiology and an understanding of basic splinting principles and of the uses and functions of hand splints are important components of the physical therapist's clinical knowledge.

The hand is a tremendously intricate, complex, and integral part of each of us. Knowledge of its intricacy leads to a greater appreciation of its beauty and versatility and to a greater empathy for the encompassing effects a hand injury can have in the lives of the patients we touch.

Be wary of technique manuals and technical compendia that attempt to match specific hand pathology to "rote" splinting. The individual problems present in the hand of each patient you treat should be thoroughly evaluated and analyzed with respect to their amenability to corrective splinting. This analytical approach should be followed as a matter of course in both the fabrication and the ongoing revision of hand splints.

In forming your own personal philosophical orientation to hand splinting in clinical practice, it is extremely important to remember a simple axiom: *Fit the splint to your patient's hand rather than attempting to fit the patient's hand to the splint.*

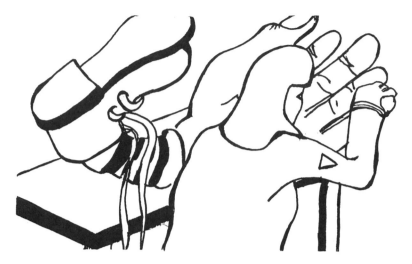

Fig. 9-1.   Avoid myopic treatment techniques.

THE HAND/UPPER EXTREMITY FUNCTIONAL UNIT:
SOME BASIC ANATOMICAL AND
KINESIOLOGICAL CONSIDERATIONS

The primary function of the hand is the ability to carry out prehensive activity (grasp, manipulation, and release of objects). The hand is responsible for the direct control of objects through the use of its intrinsic skills, but it cannot function without accurate placement by the arm. The primary role of the upper limb (shoulder, arm, elbow, and forearm) is to place the hand in its proper position of function.[1] The infinite number of objects handled and the myriad ways in which they are used make versatility the basic functional requirement of the arm.[2]

When treating the hand, it is imperative to remember that it is usually attached to a wrist, forearm, upper arm and shoulder, and to a scapula and thorax. Avoid myopic vision when treating your patients with hand injury, pathology, or dysfunction. (Fig. 9-1).

The upper extremity is suspended from the thorax, head, and neck by soft tissues. Its only point of skeletal attachment is at the sternoclavicular joint; motion in all directions is allowed by the almost flat contour of this joint. The scapula and glenohumeral joint function to provide spatial placement of the hand, with the clavicle serving as a "spanner" between the trunk and scapula, allowing motion at both the sternoclavicular and the acromioclavicular joints during shoulder elevation. Perry[2] has calculated 16,000 "arm positions" that can be attained and used for hand placement by the individual when an average of 150° of flexion, 30° of extension and 90° of abduction are present in the shoulder. Immobilization of the hand causes a decrease in the normal daily scapular and shoulder motion, and hypomobility in all joints proximal to the hand begins to occur rapidly after injury or immobilization. *Daily range of motion of all up-per extremity joints is a necessary component of a hand splinting program.*

The maximum limb length necessary for prehensile hand function is provided by extension of the elbow. With the addition of 120 to 140° of elbow flexion to the afore-mentioned average range of motion of the shoulder, Perry[2] calculates an extraordinary 2 million different possible positions for hand placement.

Pronation and supination of the forearm allow modification of hand placement in a rotatory orientation; extended immobilization of the forearm in a position other than neutral can lead to contracture of the interosseous membrane, with a resultant severe decrease in hand positioning ability.

Wrist motion aids in hand placement and in precision handling. Wrist flexion and ulnar deviation occur in combination, as do dorsiflexion and radial deviation, due to the obliquity of the wrist joints in relation to those of the hand.

OSSEOUS ANATOMY

The reader is urged to review the osseous anatomy of the wrist and hand, with em-phasis upon these palpable bony landmarks: the ulnar head, Lister's tubercle, the na-vicular and pisiform, and the metacarpal bases and heads. Brunnstrom[3] discusses the location and palpation of these landmarks in a very detailed, yet readable fashion.

HAND ARCHES

There are three structural arches in the hand, two transverse and one longitudinal arch; each contributes to hand function and dexterity.

The distal transverse metacarpal arch (Fig. 9-2) passes through the metacarpal heads; its mobility is necessary for positioning of the metacarpals during spherical grasp. (The arch deepens when a spherical object is held in the hand.) Proper func-tioning of the thumb depends upon the integrity of this arch. If the distal metacarpal arch is depressed, the hand becomes flat and the thumb is unable to carry out opposi-tion to the digits.

The longitudinal arch (Fig. 9-2) provides mobility of the digits during grasp. This arch has two components: (1) the rigid central portion, which is composed of the cen-tral carpal bone and the second and third metacarpals, and (2) completion of the arch by the other individual rays (a *ray* is defined as the metacarpal and corresponding phal-anges). Both flattening and cupping of the palm in response to objects of varying sizes are allowed by the mobility of the first, fourth, and fifth rays around the rigid second and third rays of the longitudinal arch.

The proximal transverse arch (Fig. 9-2) lies at the level of the distal carpals; its keystone is the capitate. This arch is rigid and serves to improve the mechanical advan-tage of the long finger flexors by functioning as a fulcrum to increase their leverage.

The stability and integrity of the arches are maintained by the intrinsic muscula-ture, especially the thenar and hypothenar groups. Collapse in the arch system resulting

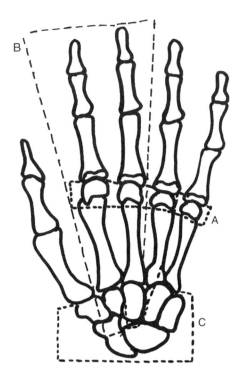

Fig. 9-2. (A) Distal transverse metacarpal; (B) longitudinal: (C) proximal transverse (carpal)

from injury to the osseous skeleton or paralysis of the intrinsic musculature can contribute to severe hand disability and deformity.[4]

MUSCULAR ANATOMY

An extensive review of anatomy of the hand musculature is disallowed by the space and scope of this chpater. For an in-depth review, the reader is guided to the following authors: Smith,[5] Wynn Parry,[6] Fess et al,[4] Cailliet,[1] Hunter et al,[7] and Brunnstrom.[3] *Surgical Anatomy of the Hand,* a CIBA publication, reprinted from *Clinical Symposia,* serves as an excellent illustrated resource in the review of anatomy of the hand.[8]

Salient points of review with which the therapist should be familiar are: (1) differentiation between intrinsic and extrinsic muscle groups; (2) origin, insertion, and innervation of each muscle; (3) an understanding of the digital extensor mechanism; and (4) a knowledge of flexor tendon sheaths and the concomitant pulley system.

In brief review, the *intrinsic muscles* are defined as "those muscles that originate within the hand and act upon the digits."[1] The thenar and hypothenar groups, the lumbricals, and the interossei are included in this definition. The extrinsics are considered to be the muscles acting on the hand whose muscle bellies originate in the forearm, proximal to the wrist joint. Although their contribution to hand function is distinctly different, the integrated function of both systems, intrinsic and extrinsic, is important to the satisfactory performance of the hand in a wide variety of tasks.[4]

The Extensor Expansion

The extensor apparatus is formed by the conjunction of the long extensor tendon, which divides at the distal end of the proximal phalanx, and the lumbricals and interossei. Its main components are the central slip and the lateral bands. The central slip attaches to the base of the middle phalanx and is stabilized at the metacarpophalangeal joint by the sagittal bands and by fibrous slips from its own volar surface. The lateral bands conjoin and insert into the distal phalanx; the bands migrate dorsally as the proximal interphalangeal joint extends. The dorsal interrosseous contributes to the formation of the extensor hood. The ulnar interosseous joins the extensor tendon on the ulnar side at the level of the head of the proximal phalanx. The lumbricals arise from the radial sides of the profundus tendons and insert into the lateral bands at the level of the proximal phalangeal heads. Distal to the site of rejoining of the lateral bands, the retinacular ligaments insert into the proximal phalanx. The reader is referred to the aforementioned authors[1,3–7] for a detailed discussion of the extensor apparatus.

With respect to intrinsic muscle function, Fess[4] states:

> an oversimplification of the function of the intrinsic musculature in the digits would be that they provide strong flexion at the metacarpophalangeal joints and extension at the proximal and distal interphalangeal joints. The lumbrical tendons, by virtue of their origin from the flexor profundi and insertion into the digital extensor mechanism, function as a governor between the two systems, resulting in a loosening of the antagonistic profundus tendon during interphalangeal joint extension.

Flexor Tendon Sheaths and Pulley System

The extrinsic flexor tendons enter the carpal tunnel beneath the deep transverse metacarpal ligament and travel through synovial sheaths on the volar side of the carpals. At approximately the level of the distal palmar crease, the profundus and superficialis divide, and the tendon slips enter digital synovial sheaths. These sheaths and their concomitant pulley system are associated with the long flexors to their points of tendon insertion. They serve as a protective housing for the tendons; their synovial lining provides a smooth gliding surface for efficient motion, and the pulleys approximate tendon to bone, thus maintaining mechanical advantage.

REVIEW OF LIGAMENTOUS ANATOMY

A listing of wrist and hand joint ligamentous anatomy is included as a brief review. The reader is referred to *Gray's Anatomy*[9] for detailed anatomical descriptions.

Radiocarpal Joint Ligaments: radial and ulnar collaterals, dorsal and palmar radiocarpal ligaments.

Intercarpal Joint Ligaments: proximal and distal row each have dorsal, volar, and interosseous ligaments that bind their respective carpals. The midcarpal joint is supported by volar, dorsal and interosseous ligaments.

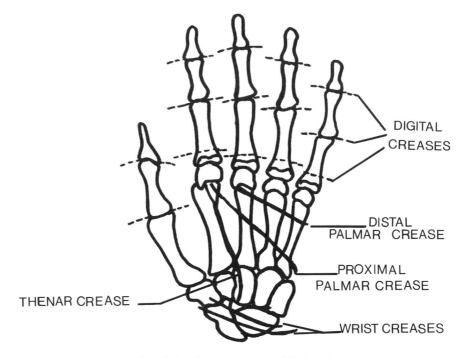

Fig. 9-3.   Flexion creases of the hand

Carpometacarpal Joints: These joints also are connected by interosseous, dorsal, and volar ligaments, while the intermetacarpal joints are connected by the transverse metacarpal ligament at their heads (metacarpals 2 to 5) and by dorsal, volar, and interosseous ligaments at their bases.

The metacarpophalangeal articulations are supported by collateral ligaments (radial and ulnar), by the palmar ligaments, and by the volar plates. This is also true for the proximal interphalangeal articulations. The distal interphalangeal joints are supported by radial and ulnar collaterals and by the palmar ligament.

FLEXION CREASES

The volar surfaces of the hand and wrist bear numerous flexion creases, which serve to allow the needed mobility of the palmar skin and soft tissue during flexion of the digits, of the thumb, and of the wrist. "Geographical" descriptions of the creases, orientation of crease positions with respect to the underlying osseous anatomy, and splinting implications will be discussed.

Digital Creases

There are three flexion creases present on the volar aspect of each digit (Fig. 9-3). The distal and the middle crease occur at the DIP and PIP joint levels, respectively, with the proximal crease located just distal to the base of the proximal phalanx. The thumb also contains three digital flexion creases, with the distal and middle creases corresponding to the same osseous structures as those of the other digits. The location of the proximal crease of the thumb occurs at the neck of the first metacarpal.

Palmar Creases

The distal palmar crease originates proximal to the head of the fifth metacarpal and curves distally to terminate between the second and third metacarpal heads. *The distal edge of dynamic and of some static splints should terminate well proximal to this crease in order to allow full flexion of the metacarpophalangeal joints.*

The proximal palmar crease originates radially just proximal to the second metacarpal head and proceeds in an ulnar direction across the palm to terminate at the hypothenar eminence.

The origin of the thenar crease is in conjunction with that of the proximal palmar crease. It curves in a proximal direction to terminate between the hypothenar and thenar eminences. The thenar crease serves as an important guideline in splint fabrication; thumb apertures should be trimmed to, or beyond, this crease in order to allow for full thumb excursion, especially opposition.

Wrist Creases

Two (sometimes three) flexion creases are present on the flexor surface of the wrist at the level of the carpals. They correspond with the wrist joint and, in the fabrication of a dynamic wrist splint, the creases are used as a guideline for location of the axes of wrist joint motion.

DUAL OBLIQUITY PRINCIPLES

The principles of dual obliquity of the hand are these: (1) the metacarpal heads demonstrate a progressive length decrease in their radial to ulnar progression and (2) the first, fourth, and fifth metacarpals exhibit a marked mobility in comparison to the rigid second and third metacarpals. Holding a pencil in the hand, with the forearm resting in a fully supinated position on a table will demonstrate these principles visually. The pencil (1) will not parallel the floor; its ulnar end will be lower than the end located on the radial side of the hand; and (2) with the wrist in a neutral (undeviated) position, the pencil will not be perpendicular to the forearm's axis, but will slant obliquely in a distal-ulnar direction from the radial to the ulnar sides of the hand.

These concepts must be incorporated into the design and fabrication of splints involving the digital metacarpals. The radial sides of these splints should be longer and higher than the ulnar border, and neither the distal edge, nor the metacarpal curve should ever be perpendicular to the long axis of the forearm.

BASIC GOALS AND PURPOSES OF HAND SPLINTING

Splinting is a viable therapeutic intervention technique in the treatment of hand injury and upper extremity dysfunction. Its uses are summarized in the following ways:

1.   Static hand splints provide *support* for painful joints (for post-operative arthrotomy patients; for the rheumatoid arthritic during "flare up" periods.)

2.   Static and dynamic hand splints aid in the *prevention of deformity* (contracture, tightness), by placing the muscles and soft tissues in as close to a functional position as possible.

3.   Splints *decrease muscle imbalance,* thus enabling weak musculature to function (a wrist-driven prehension orthosis or functional arm orthosis are examples of such devices.)

4.   *Correction* is provided through the use of specific, controlled forces (soft tissue, periarticular, and articular tightness is decreased through the stretch provided by the gradually increased force employed in a dynamic hand splint.)

5.   Splints provide the *immobilization* necessary for fracture healing and for the postoperative healing of nerve, soft tissue, and articular repairs.

6.   Static and dynamic hand splints *protect weak muscles* by disallowing their overstretch by opposing muscle groups. (They are used while awaiting return post peripheral nerve injury, after nerve graft, or following tendon or nerve repair.)

7.   The use of preoperative and postoperative splints aids in *mobilizing joints* and *strengthening musculature* through the use of constant forces transferred to the tissues through the use of outriggers, rubber bands, and finger slings.

Static Splinting

Static splints are splints that incorporate no moving parts in their design or function. They are used to provide protection, (for example, after soft tissue injury), support (use of a cock up splint), or immobilization (post-fracture or surgical repair procedures). A static splint should always hold the hand and wrist in as close to a functional position as is possible. All static splint usage should be combined with the performance of an individualized exercise program in order to prevent joint hypomobility. Specific examples of static splints are described in a later section of this chapter.

Dynamic Splinting

Dynamic splinting is the application on a moving part of a force which remains approximately constant as the part moves.[10] Traction and directional control are provided by the incorporation of finger slings, rubber bands, and outriggers into the splint design.

A second approach to dynamic splinting incorporates inherently static methods to achieve mobilization of the involved part(s). Examples of this type of splinting include serialized web spacers for the thumb, and, for the digital joints, the use of serial plaster casting or the commercial "Joint Jack" splint. Use of these types of splints facilitates increased range of motion even though the splints do not include dynamic components per se.

Dynamic splints provide constant forces over extended periods of time, while aiding in the maintenance of or facilitation of increased joint range of motion and muscle strength. The physiological benefits of dynamic splinting are: (1) joint mobility is maintained, (2) stagnant interstitial fluid and toxins are carried away, due to the

Fig. 9-4. First class lever

"pumping action" of muscle contraction, (3) tendon gliding is maintained, and (4) adhesion formation is prevented, especially of the extrinsic flexors and their digital sheaths.(5) In addition, a patient will becomes less "pain anxious" by observing to what degree he/she can actively move the involved joints with minimal discomfort.

Some basic considerations regarding the use of dynamic splinting follow:

1. Moving muscles must be given an opposing, balancing force in order to maintain joint mobility and freely gliding tendon motion. Corrective forces are supplied to carry out this goal through the utilization of outriggers, finger cuffs, and rubber bands. The strength of the rubber bands utilized should be increased gradually as gains in range of joint motion become apparent.

2. When incisions or injuries occur on the volar surface of the hand, the digits should be placed in flexion and worked into the extended position.

3. When incisions or injuries are present on the dorsal surface of the hand, splinting of the digits should be done in a neutral position and worked into the ranges of both flexion and extension.

4. The patient should be able to demonstrate the use of the dynamic splint components both for stretching and for exercise of the involved joints to the satisfaction of the therapist.

BIOMECHANICAL PRINCIPLES

Levers

Most hand/forearm splints can be considered to function as first class lever systems. The fulcrum occurs at the wrist, the forearm trough operates as the force arm (FA), and the palmar pan functions as the resistance arm, (RA) (Fig. 9-4).

The principle of mechanical advantage (MA) of a lever refers to the relationship between the length of the force arm and that of the resistance arm. In equation form this is written as: $MA = FA/RA$, meaning that either an increase in the length of the force arm or a decrease in the length of the resistance arm will result in greater mechanical advantage of the lever. This is a very important concept for incorporation into the design and fitting of hand splints. The equation becomes clinically significant, for example, when one considers a splint's palmar pan. A palmar splint component that is too short will cause an increase of pressure in the palm, with resultant patient discomfort. Lengthening of the palmar pan will decrease the possibility of this occurrence. Similarly, the longer the forearm trough, (remembering that optimum length is two-thirds of the length of the forearm), the smaller the forces present on the forearm.

Forces

Force is defined as a vector quantity that tends to produce acceleration of a body in the direction of its application. It is important to understand the practical aspects of the application of forces in splinting.

The force applied in dynamic finger traction has two components, a *rotational element* which causes joint rotation, and a *translational element* which produces either compression or distraction of the joint.[4] At the position of a 90° angle, the rotational force is at its strongest point, and the translational force is markedly decreased. In clinical terms, this principle is realized by the application of dynamic traction elements at a 90° angle of pull to the splinted part, in order to use the rotational force available and to decrease compression or distraction of the joint involved. Finger slings must be applied according to this principle for the duration of splint usage; this will entail *ongoing assessment and numerous* adjustments of the dynamic components of the splint.

Pressure

Pressure (P) is an important conceptual consideration in the practice of hand splinting. The equation, $P = F/A$ has special significance in utilization of the sustained pressures required in dynamic splinting. In practical terms, one must remember that the width of the splint strap or finger sling is very important. According to the formula, the wider the splint strap or finger sling, (A), the lower the pressure applied to the underlying tissue. This principle also applies to areas of pressure that develop over bony prominences; relief of these areas through heating and remolding of the thermoplastic material will be discussed in "Principles of Fabrication" at a later point in this chapter.

A further consideration with respect to pressure is that a finger sling should not be allowed to become tilted on the digit, thus exerting pull in a distorted position. As can be seen in the equation, $P = F/A$, as the area of contact (A) becomes smaller, the amount of force (F) exerted increases.

Three Point Pressure System

As stated earlier, a hand/forearm splint functions as a first class lever system. The forces involved function as follows: the proximal and distal ends of the splint serve as counterforces to the opposing middle force, which is supplied, usually, by the strap across the dorsum of the wrist. The hand/forearm splint is used as an example only; in all splint designs, the two parallel forces always require opposition by a middle force. These *three points of pressure* are always required for the provision of balanced forces in splinting.

SPLINTING MATERIALS

Types of Materials

The splinting materials available to the practicing therapist have evolved to include those that can be categorized as (1) high temperature plastics, (2) low temperature thermoplastics, and (3) materials whose use does not require a source of heat.

High temperature materials require a mold for formation, due to the degree of temperature necessary to obtain malleability. Two commonly used high temperature materials are Kydex and Plexiglas.

Plaster of Paris is a "no heat needed" material; its uses include serial casting of individual digits[6,11] or of the wrist and postoperative immobilization of the hand. The plaster may be used either alone, as a static splint, or as a static base to which an outrigger fashioned from the same material is attached to provide dynamic digital traction.

The low temperature thermoplastic materials are the most popular due to the facts that they are easily heated, conform to hand contours very well, and are cosmetically acceptable to the patient. The materials most commonly used are Orthoplast, Aquaplast, Polyform, and Kay-Splint. The forming temperatures for these materials may be obtained by using either wet or dry heat sources, (hydrocollator, electric skillet, or heat gun); the general range of working temperatures is from 140 to 170°. For a further discussion of materials, see Kiel,[12] or Fess.[4] A listing of splinting materials and their supply sources is included at the end of the chapter.

Splint Closures

Splint closure materials include Velcro tapes (both non-adhesive and adhesive-backed), webbing, Betapile, Vel Foam, and Soft Touch Vel-Foam. Velcro tape must be attached to the splint with adhesive compound or rivets. It is a very long-wearing closure. Betapile and Vel Foam both come in the form of polyfoam strips laminated on both sides with a soft nylon fabric. These two coverings adhere well to Velcro tape attached to the body of the splint; however, with long-term use, this ability is lessened and the straps must be replaced. Additional benefits are that patients like the softness of the material and, because of its softness, the material does not cause circumferential constriction of the forearm with resultant edema. Soft Touch Vel Foam is a new improved version of Vel Foam whose surface covering has been modified to increase its wearing life. Duravel is a similar strapping material with increased durability.

Splinting Equipment

The fabrication of hand splints requires the routine use of some specialized equipment and materials. In general, the therapist must have available a heat source, scissors, adhesives, carpentry tools, rubber bands, moleskin, Ace[12] bandages, spray coolant, rivets and eyelets and their respective setters. A listing of basic equipment and supply sources is included at the end of the chapter.

SPLINT DESIGN, FABRICATION, AND FITTING

Task Analysis Approach

Task analysis utilizes a systematic approach to problem solving. Its basic tenets can easily be utilized in evaluation of hand injury for splinting intervention and will save the therapist many undue "false starts" and "wrong turns." Kemp[13] delineates three essential elements of this systems approach with respect to instructional design.

Transposed for use in splinting assessment, these basic questions are: (1) what must be accomplished?, (2) what methods will work best to reach the desired goal(s)?, and (3) how will it be known that the goal has been reached?

If the answers to these questions reveal a splinting need, the problems to be addressed should be ranked according to their degree of importance; primary, secondary, and associated problems should be included. Once these problems have been ranked, one may progress in a questioning hierarchy. The following sequence is a suggested one:

1. Identification of primary, secondary, and associated problems.
2. What do I expect to accomplish through the use of a splint?
3. What splint components are integral to correction of the problems?
4. What splint design will best encompass these components?
5. Should the splint be static or dynamic?
6. Should the base be volar or dorsal?
7. What joints should be included in the splint?
8. What is the patient's level of cognition? Is it adequate for correct wearing and usage of the splint?
9. What is the patient's emotional status?

In defining the problems to be addressed in rehabilitation of the patient with a hand injury, it should be recognized that psychological, emotional, and vocational factors all have a bearing and an impact upon treatment outcomes. Especially important is recognition of the psychological aspects of hand injury. These are myriad and one must be cognizant of the fact that they can be of greater importance in the patient's life than all of the physical intervention provided by the medical team. The literature does not contain a voluminous amount of information regarding this aspect of hand rehabilitation. Pulvertaft[14] addresses his comments to surgeons on possible psychological problems associated with hand injury. These include causalgia, malingering, hysteria, and difficulties encountered in cases of self-inflicted injuries. Wynn Parry[6] addresses the psychological problems of upper extremity amputees.

The work of Shontz[15] and of Wright[16] are both highly recommended to the reader for expanded discussions of the psychological aspects of physical disability. The basic principles addressed in these two works apply most directly to the treatment of the hand-injured patient.

PRINCIPLES OF FABRICATION

Pattern Design and Material Selection

Pattern-making is an integral part of the splint fabrication process, especially for therapists new to splint design or for therapists who are not involved with splinting as a daily part of their clinical practice.

A pattern should be designed and made for each individual splint. Just as a commercially pre-fabricated splint is not designed for each specific patient, neither should a commercial pattern be seen as the standard answer for beginning the process of fabrication of a hand splint. Commercial patterns are best used as guidelines for determining the general shape or outline of a splint.

When formulating a pattern, it is expedient to use a soft, pliable, absorbent material that is inexpensive; paper towels, tissue paper, and soft cotton are materials that work well. Plastic wrap is very useful for visualization of the underlying tissues while drawing the pattern. Exposed x-ray film is another material utilized by some therapists for pattern design. Using a marking pen, follow the anatomical outlines of the hand and forearm. Allow ample room for the rolling and contouring of splint edges and for adequate support of the part, especially with respect to the ulnar and radial sides of a forearm trough. The reader is referred to Fess[4] and to Kiel[12] for a thorough discussion of pattern design.

Transfer of the pattern to the appropriate splinting material should be done using an awl or lead pencil; these marks will not appear on the finished splint, as will those made by the use of a felt tip marker or of a ball point pen.

Working With the Material: Practical Clinical Procedures and Information

As the splint design and fabrication process is begun, the patient should be seated for design of the pattern with the forearm and hand resting on a table that is a comfortable height for both patient and therapist. Materials and equipment should be arranged together in a central "work area" close to the patient, thus decreasing the amount of unnecessary leg work on the part of the therapist.

Once the pattern has been designed, transferred to the appropriate material, and cut out, the patient's forearm and hand should be positioned in the anti-gravity position with his/her elbow resting on the table. Foam padding under the elbow makes this position more comfortable for the patient; this position is also a very good one for ease of operation for the therapist.

The warmed splinting material should be molded to the hand, wrist, and forearm, working in a distal to proximal direction to assure correct fit of the digital, thumb, and arch components of the splint. The wrist is molded next, positioning it in the correct amount of dorsiflexion, and the forearm is correctly positioned in the trough. During the forming of this splint component, one should be careful to avoid supination of the forearm, thus causing it to migrate out of the splint. The splint is held in position with Ace wraps or other smooth, wide, elastic material while the material hardens. This setting process may be facilitated through the use of a spray coolant.

When the material has hardened, trim lines are drawn and excess material cut away; the splint should then be softened again and remolded to the hand and forearm. While this procedure may seem tedious and time-consuming, the second remolding process yields a smooth, correct fit, and reduces the need for numerous revisions and involved trimming of the final product. Proper fit of the splint should be assessed with respect to the following components: (1) all edges must be smooth (either rolled or adequately trimmed), (2) hand arches should be correctly placed and incorporated into the palmar pan of the splint, and (3) the thumb must be allowed adequate room for excursion. In addition, the splint must be checked for pressure points over the bony prominences of the hand and wrist. If these are present, they must be heated and relieved to decrease the potential of skin maceration or pressure sore formation. *Note:* these areas should be relieved rather than padded, as the overzealous use of padding will distort the design and the proper fit of the splint, and may cause a pressure increase over the bony prominence. Additional considerations are that the length of the forearm trough of a splint should measure two-thirds of the length of the patient's forearm in order to allow unimpeded elbow flexion and extension. The height of the radial and ulnar sides of the trough should bisect the forearm on its respective medial and lateral sides.

Dynamic Components

Dynamic components (outriggers, finger slings, and rubber bands) are attached to the static splint base. Outriggers may be fabricated from splinting materials, wire, banding material, or welding rod. Moleskin, Elastikon tape, felt, or leather are materials utilized for fabrication of finger slings. When attaching slings, the rotational forces acting upon the digits must be carefully considered; *repeated on-going adjustments are required as the range of motion of the digits changes.* One means of assuring the correct direction of digital rotation is to attach the adhesive surface of the moleskin sling directly to the skin of the finger, rather than lining the sling with a second layer of moleskin.[17] The sling is then used to rotate the digit in the corrected position.

Straps and Closures

Straps and closures should be attached securely to the splint. They should be positioned to maintain the hand and foearm in the correct positions; in the case of a hand/wrist splint incorporating a forearm trough, the straps include a proximal attachment, one positioned over the dorsum of the wrist, and a third strap over the dorsal aspect of the digits. Remember that $P = F/A$; therefore, to decrease pressure on soft tissues and bony prominences, increase the width of the straps. Straps over the dorsum of the hand and wrist should be wide and soft in order to avoid compromising the venous blood flow, which causes resultant edema formation.

The *cosmesis* of a splint is an integral element in patient compliance with the prescribed program of wear and also serves as a professional reflection upon the therapist. This fact cannot be overstressed, especially in the era of professional accountability and cost effectiveness. Repeated practice with materials and designs is essential to the development of a therapist's skill, competence, and confidence in the process of splint fabrication.

Patient Education

Instruction of the patient in correct splint wearing and usage is one of the most crucial aspects of a hand splinting program. The therapist should teach the patient: (1) how to apply and remove the splint, including its dynamic components; (2) how the dynamic splint is to be used as an exercise device; (3) how often a static splint must be removed for active or passive exercise of the hand, (4) how and where to check the hand and forearm for possible development of pressure areas, and (5) the correct exercise program to be performed. The patient should be able to demonstrate these five procedures to the satisfaction of the therapist. If the patient's cognitive ability is such that this is not possible, a family member or significant other person should be so instructed.

Written instructions with clear illustrations regarding splint usage and an individualized exercise program should *always* be a part of patient education in a hand rehabilitation program. The use of written "handouts" is very beneficial in clinical practice. Handouts serve to: (1) organize patient information, (2) standardize basic theoretical information (i.e., warning signs: edema, pain, pressure areas, numbness, tingling), (3) provide a basis for your attesting to the information received by the patient, and (4) minimize the problem of giving ineffective patient instruction due to time limitations.[18]

TYPES OF SPLINTS

Because each therapist employs his or her own personal approach to hand splinting, there are myriad ways of approaching the design and fabrication of individual splints. The following section contains a discussion of selected static and dynamic splints, along with some of the more frequently encountered problems and situations in which their use is appropriate. It should be noted that these splints are not to be considered as universal answers, but rather are suggested as possible means of intervention in the treatment of hand injuries.

As discussed earlier in this chapter, the use of commercially fabricated splints should be considered very judiciously and their use implemented only after careful evaluation and assessment of the problems involved. Modifications and adjustments of these splints for the individual patient are *always* required. To quote Malick,[10] "a splint that fits everyone fits no one."

Custom-Designed and Fabricated Static Splints

1. Anti-Swan Neck Splint. This is a simple splint used to prevent hyperextension of the proximal interphalangeal joint, which can be easily fabricated from a small piece of thermoplastic material (Fig. 9-5). The joint is positioned in 10° of flexion; the splint does not interfere with prehensile hand function, yet prevents progression of the deformity through daily use and night wearing.

2. Anti-Boutonniere Splint. This simple splint may be fabricated from thermoplastic material and used to decrease the progression of boutonnière deformity of the proximal interphalangeal joint. In essence, it is a reverse of the anti-swan neck splint (Fig. 9-6).

3. Opponens Splint. The use of an opponens, or thumb web space splint, offers an extremely beneficial means of increasing or maintaining the web space of the thumb. This splint is easily contoured to the thumb, the web space, and the hand through the use of low temperature material; it should be designed to hold the thumb in a position of maximum available opposition (Fig. 9-7). These splints may be used in serial form,[4,19] through the fabrication of sequential, modified splints, as increases in web

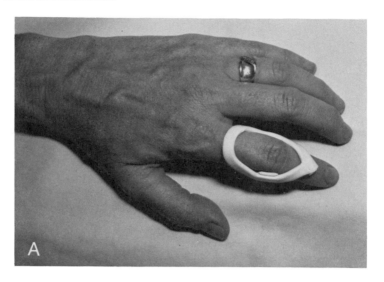

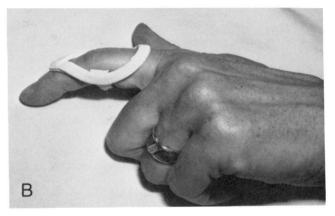

Fig. 9-5.   Anti-Swan neck splints (Courtesy of Judith M. Hansan, R.P.T., Wichita, Kansas)

space measurements are apparent. As a review of the mechanism of contracture of the thumb web space, the reader is referred to Phelps and Weeks.[20]

4. Safe Position Splint (Burn Splint). This static splint serves as a positioning device during healing of the burned hand.[21] The aspects of joint positioning unique to this splint are: (a) the metacarpophalangeal joints are placed in 90° of flexion, and (b) the proximal and distal interphalangeal joints are positioned in full extension. This specialized positioning serves to maintain collateral ligament lengths at the metacarpophalangeal and interphalangeal joints and to prevent development of the "intrinsic minus" deformity. In addition, the thumb should be positioned to maintain full passive range of motion of the first carpometacarpal joint. The optimum wrist position is 30° of dorsiflexion. This may need to be obtained gradually, however. Use of the safe position splint is in conjunction with a strict exercise regimen; its wearing decreases from 24 hour use to night use only, as the healing progresses (Fig. 9-8).

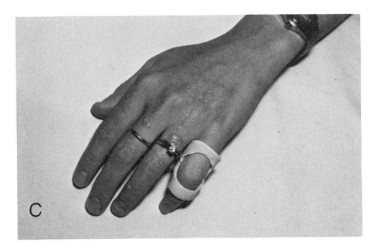

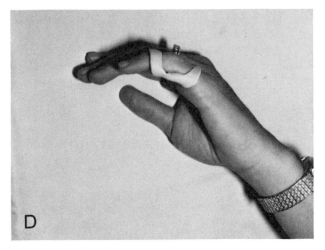

Fig. 9-5.   *(cont.)*

5. Functional Position Splint. The use of a functional position splint is indicated when immobilization of the hand and wrist are required (Fig. 9-9). Conditions in which the use of such a splint may prove valuable are after corrective surgical procedures (trauma, capsulotomy, fracture pinning, arthrotomy), and during the "flare up" periods experienced by the patient with rheumatoid arthritis. Joint positions to be incorporated into a functional position splint are 25 to 30° of wrist dorsiflexion, and flexion of meta-carpophalangeal and interphalangeal joints of 40 to 45°, with the thumb positioned in abduction and opposition, its pad lined up with the pads of the digits.

6. Wrist Cock Up Splint. This static splint serves the function of maintaining wrist dorsiflexion (extension) while allowing prehensile function of the fingers and thumb (Fig. 9-10). It is useful in cases of weakness of the wrist extensors or extrinsic finger extensors and at times when extra wrist and palmar arch support are required for the fa-

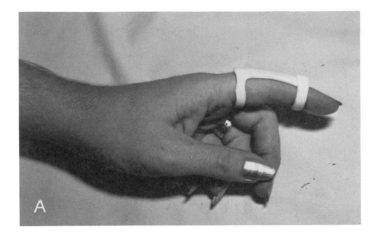

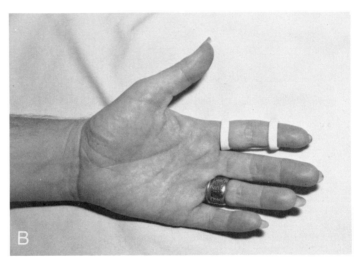

Fig. 9-6. Anti-boutonniere split (Courtesy of Judith M. Hansan, R.P.T., Wichita, Kansas)

cilitation of hand function. Increase wrist dorsiflexion to 25 to 30° as allowed by progression in range of motion.

7. Spasticity Reduction Splints. Much controversy exists regarding the use of splinting in treatment of the hand exhibiting hypertonus. Much of this controversy revolves around the benefits of a volarly versus a dorsally based splint.[22–27] Snook[26] has designed what is essentially a dorsally-based static splint which aids markedly in reduction of tone in the spastic hand. McPherson et al[27] evaluated both dorsal-based and volar-based splints and concluded that both served to reduce hypertonicity. Younger subjects (35 years of age and younger) demonstrated a significant decline in tone in comparison with patients over age 65, who demonstrated a gradual, but not significant reduction of hypertonicity.

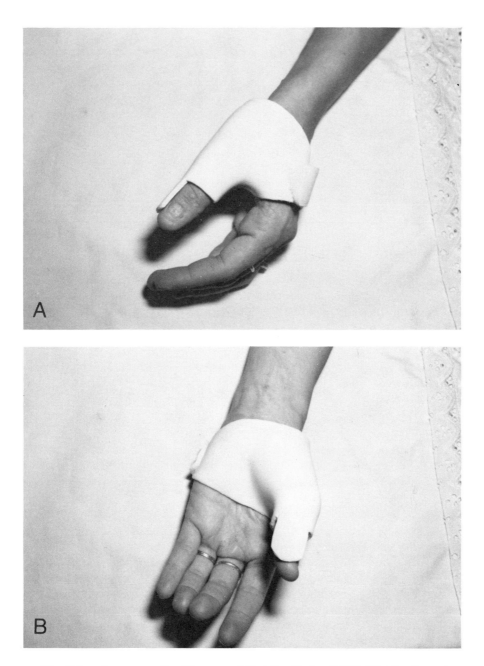

Fig. 9-7.   Opponens splint (Courtesy of Christine Statler, R.P.T, Wichita, Kansas)

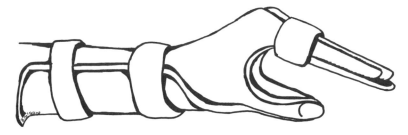

Fig. 9-8. Safe postition splint

For further theoretical consideration, the reader is referred to an interesting survey of 93 occupational therapists regarding their personal rationales regarding splinting of the hemiplegic hand.[28]

Commercially Made Static Splints

Alumafoam Alumafoam is a versatile splinting material that is available in the form of lightweight aluminum strips backed on one side with soft foam rubber. The strips come in standard lengths, but in a variety of widths. The amount of material

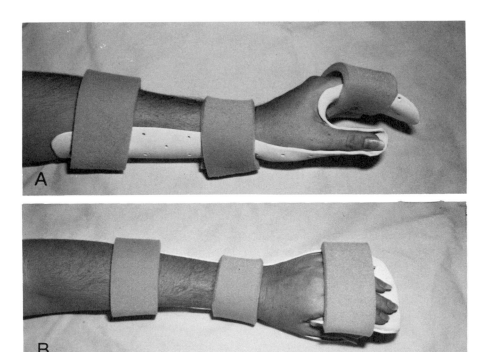

Fig. 9-9. Functional position splint (Courtesy of Harold Calkins, C.P.O., Phoenix, Arizona)

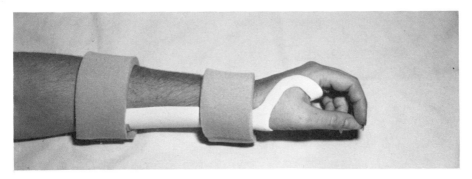

Fig. 9-10. Cock up splint (Courtesy of Harold Calkins, C.P.O., Phoenix, Arizona)

needed for immobilization of the joint is measured and cut from the strip and then taped in its correct position, on either the volar or the dorsal surface of the digit (Fig. 9-11). This type of static splinting is easy and quick to perform, is inexpensive, and generally has good patient compliance.

Alumafoam is a useful splinting mode for use in the treatment of proximal interphalangeal joint problems (boutonnière or swan neck deformities) and in distal interphalangeal joint pathology (mallet finger or terminal extensor tendon avulsion). This type of static splinting is indicated also for selective immobilization of joints when one is attempting to direct forces to a specific joint movement. Examples are immobilization of the digital interphalangeal joints in extension to facilitate intrinsic motion at the metacarpophalangeal joints or immobilization of the thumb metacarpophalangeal joint to facilitate use of the long thumb flexor and extensor at the interphalangeal joint.

"Joint Jack" This splint is useful in treatment of flexion contractures of the proximal interphalangeal joint. This lightweight, malleable, steel splint is padded with felt and incorporates a volar screw which is adjusted to maintain the desired amount of stretch on the joint and the corrected joint position (Fig. 9-12).

Great care and diligence are required in the utilization of this splint, as incorrect or overzealous stretching will lead to the development of pressure necrosis or to tendon rupture. When attempting to ameliorate a flexion contracture of the proximal interphalangeal joint, the advantages of using this splint must be weighed carefully over those of the individually fabricated dynamic PIP extension splint.

Custom-Fabricated Dynamic Splints

Wrist Flexion/Extension Splint Functional wrist motion, especially dorsiflexion, is integral to hand function. The use of a dynamic wrist flexion/extension splint provides an efficacious means of attaining and/or maintaining this necessary motion.

Construction of a dynamic wrist splint entails the fabrication of a static palmar pan/forearm trough which is then cut and hinged at the axis of the wrist joint to allow active and actively-assisted flexion and extension of the wrist. Volar and/or dorsal outriggers are attached, as indicated, and rubber bands of graduated strengths are used to

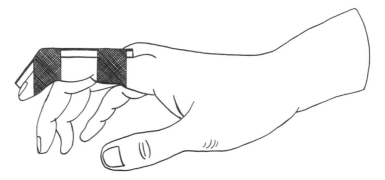

Fig. 9-11.   Alumafoam technique

supply the dynamic component. Dynamic wrist splints may be fabricated in low profile form,[29] or with outriggers of conventional design (Fig. 9-13).

   The use of a dynamic wrist flexion/extension splint is beneficial in the maintenance of wrist range of motion following wrist arthroplasty procedures[30] and after tendon repair or surgical tenolysis.

   Metacarpophalangeal Joint Flexion/Extension Splint This dynamic splint provides assistance or resistance to flexion or extension, or to both motions, as indicated by the evaluated needs (Fig. 9-14). Outriggers may be positioned on either the volar or the dorsal aspects of the static base; most often both are included in the splint design. Individual slings and rubber bands of graduated strengths are used for correct digital alignment. Slings are applied to the proximal phalanges of the involved digits. Alignments in the desired direction and in the degree of deviation must be incorporated into the positioning of the slings, both on the digits and on the outriggers. Ongoing adjustment of the dynamic components are indicated as increases in the metacarpophalangeal joint range of motion are assessed. Outriggers and slings must be observed and adjusted to maintain the necessary 90° angle of pull on the proximal phalanx.

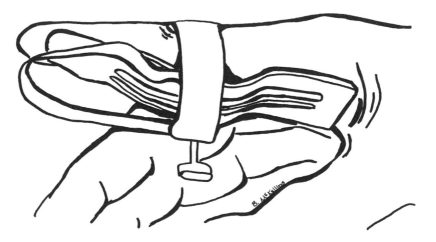

Fig. 9-12.   "Joint Jack" splint

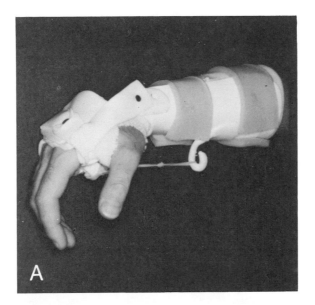

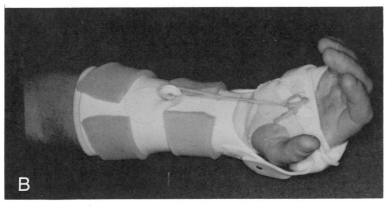

Fig. 9-13. Low profile wrist flexion splint (Courtesy of Christine Muhleman, O.T.R. and Gloria De Vore, O.T.R., Tucson, Arizona)

The most frequent indication for this type of dynamic splinting is following metacarpophalangeal arthroplasty procedures.[31,32] It is also useful following extensor tendon repair and after soft tissue injury or repair.

Proximal Interphalangeal Joint Flexion/Extension Splint This type of splint design is indicated when mobilization of the proximal interphalangeal joint is the desired therapeutic goal (Fig. 9-15).

The splint design must incorporate a provision for immobilization of the metacarpophalangeal joint and proximal phalanx, in order to prevent diversion of the active extension force to this joint from its intended target. The extension outrigger is designed for the involved digit to provide both a dynamic extension force to the middle phalanx and graded resistance for motion of the extrinsic finger flexors. The flexion force is di-

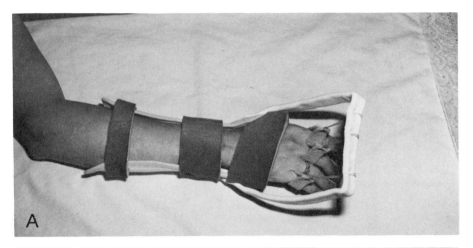

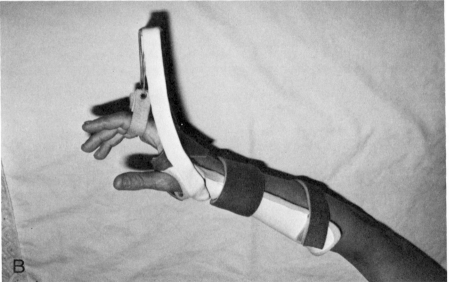

Fig. 9-14.   Dynamic MCP flexion splint

rected to the proximal interphalangeal joint through the use of a finger cuff attached to a segment of nylon line and rubber band of the appropriate required strength. The nylon line maintains its specific digital alignment by passing through a small grommet or eyelet correctly positioned in the palmar pan.

The use of this type of dynamic splint is indicated after flexor or extensor tendon repair or following proximal interphalangeal joint arthroplasty procedures. As is true with other types of dynamic hand splints, this particular splint may be fabricated as a conventional or as a low profile design.

"Finger Trapper" or "Buddy System" Splint The "buddy system" splint fits the category of dynamic splinting in that it utilizes the active force of one digit to aid in the mobilization of the joints of the adjacent digit (Fig. 9-16). This splint is useful following phalangeal fracture, soft tissue injury, or joint pathology. It is also beneficial in the treatment of the "pain anxious" patient who requires the visual and proprioceptive reassurance and feedback supplied by such an assistive device for increasing digital range of motion.

Dynamic Thumb Splints Most dynamic thumb splints utilize forces to aid in the mobilization of the metacarpophalangeal or interphalangeal joints in the motions of flexion or extension. A contiguous fit is assured when these splints are fabricated from one of the low temperature thermoplastic materials (Fig. 9-17). A dynamic thumb splint should place the thumb in an opposed position, maintain the web space and palmar arch, and allow unimpeded wrist motion, especially radial deviation. In fitting a dynamic thumb splint to allow flexion of the interphalangeal joint, one must remember to trim the distal volar edge well below the distal flexion crease to allow unrestricted motion of the long flexor tendon at this joint.

Commercially Fabricated Dynamic Splints

"Capener" Splint This commercially available splint is designed to aid in the reduction of proximal interphalangeal joint flexion contractures. It is made of thin gauge wire coiled at the axis of the proximal interphalangeal joint, with a proximal volar metacarpophalangeal pad, a dorsal pad on the proximal phalanx, and a distal strap for stabilization of the splint upon the digit (Fig. 9-18).

As with other commercial splints, adjustments of this splint are necessary, usually in the length or in the joint axis placement. One can facilitate patient comfort and wearing of the splint by beginning splint usage with short periods of wearing time and loosening of the distal strap. Wearing time intervals are steadily increased, and the distal strap is successively shortened so that the splint will correctly conform to the digit and provide adequate extension force on the proximal interphalangeal joint.

FURTHER RESOURCES

The therapist who wishes further information on the subject of hand splinting principles and design is referred to The American Society of Hand Therapists. This professional organization serves as an excellent resource for the provision of reference materials, a research bibliography, and resource persons with expertise in the area of hand rehabilitation.

Materials List

1. Kydex-Rohm & Haas Independence Mall West Philadelphia, PA 19105
2. Plexiglas-Rohm & Haas
3. Orthoplast-Johnson & Johnson Co. 501 George St. New Brunswick, New Jersey 08903
4. Aquaplast-WFR/Aquaplast Corp. P.O. Box 215 Ramsey, New Jersey 07446

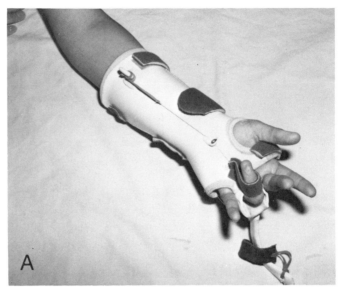

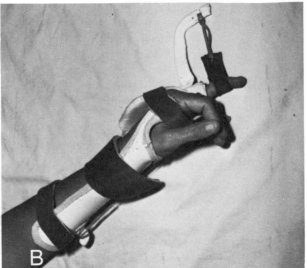

Fig. 9-15.   (A,B) Dynamic PIP flexion/extension splint

    5. Polyform Ezeform-Rolyan Medical Products 14475 Whittaker Way P.O. Box 555 Menomonee Fals, Wisconsin 53051

    6. Kay-Splint-Fred Sammons Co., Inc. P.O. Box 32 Brookfield, Illinois

    7. Velcro Tape-Fred Sammons Co., Inc.

    8. Betapile-Ali-Med, Inc. 138 Prince Street Boston, Mass. 03113

    9. Vel Foam-Fred Sammons Co., Inc.

    10. Soft Touch Vel Foam-Fred Sammons Co., Inc.

    11. Duravel-WFR/Aquaplast Corp.-Hand Rehab Products, Inc. Dept. 101, P.O. 5442 Compton, California 90224

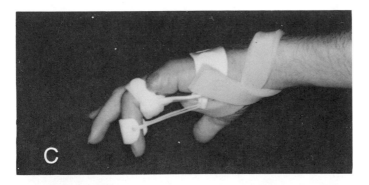

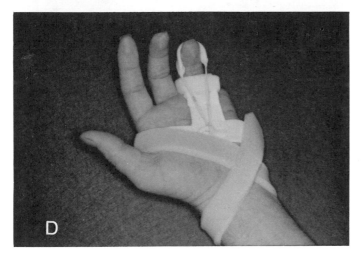

Fig. 9-15 (*cont.*) (C,D) Low profile dynamic PIP flexion/extension splint (Courtesy of Christina Muhleman, O.T.R. & Gloria De Vore, O.T.R., Tucson, Arizona)

12. Ace Bandages-Local medical supply house Local pharmacy
13. Elastikon-Johnson & Johnson Co.
14. Alumaform-Conco Chemical Co. 380 Horace St. Bridgeport, Conn. 06610
15. Plaster of Paris-Local medical supply company

Splinting Supplies

1. Heat source: Hydrocollator or electric skillet
2. Heat gun
3. Linoleum knife
4. Scissors: curved blade splinting and bandage or meniscus
5. Ace bandages
6. Leather punch
7. Rivet setter and rivets (alloy—not brass as they are affected by perspiration and they tend to "work loose" when used in low temperature materials)

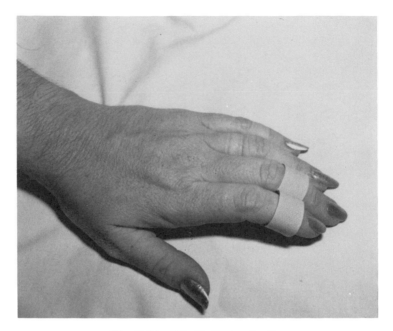

Fig. 9-16.   "Buddy System" splint

8. Eyelet setter and eyelets
9. Terry cloth towels
10. Cold spray (for quick setting of low temperature thermoplastics).
11. Ice water (works well for rapid hardening of the entire splint).

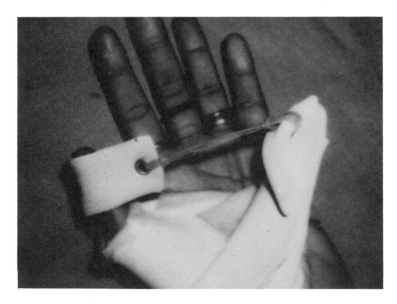

Fig. 9-17.   Dynamic Thumb IP flexion splint

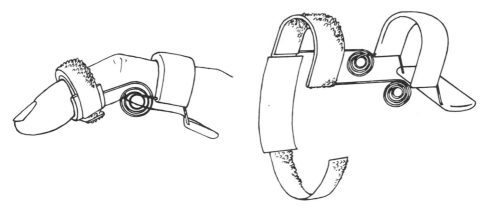

Fig. 9-18. "Capener" splint

12. Rubber bands (graduated strengths)
13. Velcro (both hook and pile for fastening)
14. Moleskin brand adhesive lining material
15. Vise
16. Pliers
17. Hammer
18. Sand paper
19. Compression foam
20. Leather (for finger slings)
21. Elastikon brand tape (for finishing edges, for making finger slings, and for attaching aluminum finger splints).
22. Dress hooks and Super Glue or other bonding material (for fingernail traction).
23. Silicone foam elastomer (for use in making post-graft burn splints and for maintaining digital alignment in resting splints).
24. Alumafoam brand splinting strips

SUMMARY

Splinting is a dynamic, continually evolving art, a viable component in the treatment of patients with hand injuries and upper extremity dysfunction. The evolution and improvement of splinting materials and equipment has aided therapists in the fabrication of affordable, better fitting, and more cosmetically acceptable splints than have ever been possible previously.

Splint design and fabrication are skills that improve with continued exercise. Physical therapists must accept the challenge of learning, relearning, synthesizing, and re-evaluating their knowledge of upper extremity anatomy and kinesiology, and of splinting principles and techniques, in order to deliver the highest quality of care possible to those hand-injured patients whose lives we touch.

ACKNOWLEDGMENTS

The author gratefully acknowledges the assistance of the following persons without whose support and encouragement this chapter would not have been possible: Christine Muhleman, OTR, Christine Statler, RPT, Harold Calkins, CPO, Judith M. Hansan, RPT, Brenda Mc Kellips, Belinda Harness, and Irene King. A special thanks to John Gribben, for his ongoing support and belief in this work.

REFERENCES

1. Cailliet R: Hand pain and impairment. 2nd Ed. FA Davis Co, Philadelphia, 1975
2. Perry J: Normal upper extremity kinesiology. Phys Ther 58:3, 1978
3. Brunnstrom S: Clinical kinesiology. 3rd Ed FA Davis Co, Philadelphia, 1972
4. Fess E, Gettle K, Strickland J: Hand splinting: principles and methods. CV Mosby Co, St Louis, 1981
5. Smith R: Intrinsic muscles of the fingers: function, dysfunction, and surgical reconstruction. American Academy of Orthopedic Surgeons: Instructional Course Lectures, 1975
6. Wynn Parry, CB: Rehabilitation of the hand. 4th Ed. Butterworths, London, 1981
7. Hunter J, Schneider L, Mackin E, Bell J: Rehabilitation of the hand. CV Mosby Co, St Louis, 1978
8. Lampe EW: Surgical anatomy of the hand. CIBA, reprinted from Clin Symp 21:3, 1969
9. Gray H: Anatomy of the human body. 28th ed. Goss CM (ed): Lea & Febiger, Philadelphia,1966
10. Malick M: Manual on static hand splinting: new materials and techniques. Rev. Ed. Harmarville Rehabilitation Center, Pittsburg, 1972
11. Bell J: Plaster cylinder casting of contractures of the interphalangeal joints. In Hunter JM et al: Rehabilitation of the hand. CV Mosby Co, St Louis, 1978
12. Kiel J: Basic hand splinting: a pattern-designing approach. Little, Brown and Co, Boston, 1983
13. Kemp JE: Instructional design: a plan for unit and course development. 2nd Ed. Fearon-Pitman, Belmont, CA 1977
14. Pulvertaft RG: Psychological aspects of hand injuries. In Hunter JM et al: Rehabilitation of the hand. CV Mosby Co, St Louis, 1978
15. Shontz FC: The psychological aspects of physical illness and disability. Macmillan, New York, 1975
16. Wright BA: Physical disability—a psychological approach. Harper and Row, New York, 1960
17. Muhleman C: Personal communication, 1983
18. Freedman CR: Teaching patients. Courseware, San Diego, 1978
19. Fess EE: Splinting for mobilization of the thumb. In Hunter et al: Rehabilitation of the hand. CV Mosby Co, St Louis, 1978
20. Phelps P, Weeks P: Management of the thumb-index web space contracture. Am J Occup Ther 30:9, 1976
21. Von Prince K, Yeakel M: The splinting of burn patients. Charles C. Thomas, Springfield, 1974
22. Kaplan N: Effects of sensorimotor stimulation in treatment of spasticity. Arch Phys Med 43, 1962
23. Gillette H: The treatment of cerebral palsy. Phys Ther Rev 32, 1952

24. Chariat S: A comparison of volar and dorsal splinting of the hemiplegic hand. Am J Occup Ther 22, 1968
25. Farber S, Huss J: Sensorimotor evaluation and treatment procedures for allied health personnel. Indiana University, Purdue University—Indianapolis Medical Center, Indianapolis, 1974
26. Snook J: Spasticity reduction splint. Am J Occup Ther 33, 1979
27. McPherson J, Kreimeyer D, Aalderks M, Gallagher T: A comparison of dorsal and volar resting hand splints in the reduction of hypertonus. Am J Occup Ther 36, 1982
28. Neuhaus B, Ascher E, Coullon B et al: A survey of rationales for and against hand splinting in hemiplegia. Am J Occup Ther 35, 1981
29. Colditz J: Low profile dynamic splinting of the injured hand. Am J Occup Ther 37, 1983
30. Johnson B, Flynn MJ, Beckenbaugh RJ: A Dynamic Splint for use after total wrist arthroplasty. Am J Occup Ther 35, 1981
31. Gribben M, Gabbert MJ, Hansan J, Muhleman C: Metacarpophalangeal arthroplasty: a case report. Phys Ther 61, 1981
32. Carter M, Wilson R: Postsurgical management in rheumatoid arthritis. In Hunter JM et al: Rehabilitation of the hand. CV Mosby, St Louis, 1978

10 | Fractures of the Wrist and Hand

Mary K. Sorenson

Fractures of the wrist and hand are relatively common injuries, and yet, if mismanaged, they can lead to significant disability and limitation in function. This chapter will be divided into subsections, discussing the basic principles of fracture management; the pathophysiology of fracture wound healing and the medical/surgical therapeutic treatment; and the complications involved in wrist fractures or dislocations, carpal fractures and dislocations, metacarpal fractures, and phalangeal fractures, respectively. There will also be a small discussion on the priorities of care with multiple fractures.

BASIC PRINCIPLES

When treating any fracture of the wrist and hand, the basic principles of fracture wound healing must be applied. These are proper diagnosis, adequate reduction of the fracture, immobilization and protection of the fracture during healing, maintenance of mobilization of all uninvolved joints, and then mobilization of the joints distal and proximal to the fracture. The foundation upon which these principles are formed is based on adequate knowledge of the biology of fracture healing. By understanding the pathophysiology of wound healing, proper choices can be made in the treatment of the fracture and the expected result of such treatment.

FRACTURE WOUND HEALING

Perhaps one of the most unique features in fracture healing is that this wound heals without a scar,[1,2] and the injured tissue is restructured by a tissue very much like its original make-up. There are several phases of bone repair that happen consecu-

191

Table 10-1. Fracture Healing Rate

Fractures of the distal radius	
Colles'	
Undisplaced	4 wk[2]
Displaced	6 wk[2] or 4–7 wk[7]
Smith's	6 wk[2]
Carpal Fractures	
Scaphoid	3 mo or more[2]
	(Need union on x-ray)
Tubercle of scaphoid	8–10 wk[7]
Hamate	4–6 wk[21]
Capitate	Needs union on x-ray[21]
Triquetrum	6 wk[21]
Metacarpal Fractures	3–5 wk[10]
Neck	3–4 wk[7,26]
Shaft	3–5 wk[31] or 4–7 wk[26]
Base	3–5 wk[10] or 4–6 wk[26]
Proximal Phalanx Fractures	
Base	3–5 wk[10]
Shaft	5–7 wk[26] or 3–4 wk[7]
Head and neck	3–5 wk[10]
Middle Phalanx Fractures	
Base	3–5 wk[10]
Shaft	10–14 wk[10,26]
Head and neck articular	3–5 wk[10]
Distal Phalanx Fractures	
Articular	3–5 wk[10] or 2 wk[7,28]
Thumb Fractures	
Bennett's	6 wk[26] or 4–6 wk[31]
Rolando	3–4 wk[26] or 4–6 wk[31]

Superscript numbers refer to references.

tively, as well as concurrently. The first phase is the *inflammatory phase*. Bleeding from the bone and surrounding soft tissue forms a fracture hematoma in which increased cellular activity begins cleaning up the debris. The bone fragment ends die and serve a passive role in the bridging process. The active bridging in the Primary Callus Response is from more distant living bone, intact periosteum, and surrounding soft tissue. This fundamental reaction to bone injury is almost independent of environmental circumstances. However, this response dies quickly if bone fragment ends do not make contact.[1]

The second phase of healing occurs from the formation of *external* and *internal callus* to bridge the gap. Osteogenic cells proliferate from both the periosteum (to form an external callus) and the endosteum (to form the internal callus), producing a tumor-like mass of irregular bone and calcified cartilage, forming a "clinical union" of the fracture. At this stage, radiographic evidence of healing is not present. A fracture is considered "clinically healed" when there is no motion at the fracture site when stressed and there is no pain at the fracture site with active movement.[2]

The final phase is the *remodeling of bone*. Cortical bone and cancellous bone differ in the process, but both involve the removal and replacement of bone throughout their respective osteoclast, osteoblast, and vascular system.[3] Blood vessels and cancellous bone are not far from the trabeculae, so bone replacement can take place on the surface of the trabeculae; this process is often referred to as "creeping substitution."[1] Osteoclasts in cortical bone need to tunnel through dead bone, bringing a blood vessel

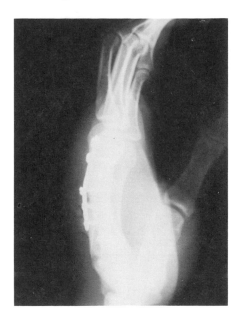

Fig. 10-1. Radiograph of bent compression plate on third metacarpal fracture 10 weeks post-fixation.

and osteoblast with it to lay down laminar bone. This remodeling process may continue for years, but radiographic union is usually seen within a few months from the time of fracture.[1,2,4] Despite all these variables, there are some general guidelines for the rate of fracture healing. See Table 10-1 as a guideline for these rates.

GENERAL GUIDELINES OF SURGICAL MANAGEMENT

Although the biological rate of fracture healing is often beyond our control, by being aware of this healing process, we can apply its clinical implications to the treatment. For example, early mobilization to prevent joint stiffness is a priority in fracture treatment, so the use of rigid internal fixation, such as the compression plate, once seemed to be an answer for this problem. Now, however, rigid immobilization is thought to suppress the external callus phase of bone healing, thus putting the stress on the fixation device until the slower bone remodelling can take place.[1] The plate then has to remain strong enough to tolerate the stresses placed on it; and, as you can see in Fig. 10-1, the device may give out before healing is complete. There is also concern that the metal fixation device, when left on for too long, can create stress protection atrophy of the bone, and therefore needs to be removed as soon as healing is seen on the fracture.[1] A new form of internal fixation now under investigation is an intramedullary fixation device with a polylactic acid polymer (PLA)-carbon fiber composite. It is capable of withstanding the bending moments in normal pinch and has several advantages over the metal internal fixation devices.[5] A most fascinating aspect is that this device over time "biologically" attaches itself to the healing bone, and thereby increases its strength and rigidity. After fracture healing is complete, the low carbon content of the device degrades almost completely, thus avoiding stress protection atrophy and the

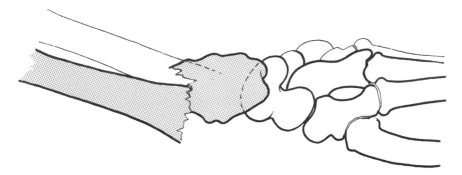

Fig. 10-2.   Colles' fracture: extra-articular fracture with dorsal displacement.

need for a second surgical procedure to remove the device.[5] If proven successful, this would certainly be a useful alternative in metacarpal and phalangeal fracture fixations.

GUIDELINES OF THERAPEUTIC MANAGEMENT

The basic principles of treating all fractures in the hand and wrist are essentially the same, though there are 30 bones which could fracture at different sites, angles, and degrees of complexities. Proper diagnosis of the fracture/fractures is made through clinical observation, complete history of the injury, full x-ray (AP, lateral and oblique), and analysis of the soft tissue injury accompanying the fracture. After a diagnosis is made, the fracture may need to be reduced by means of closed reduction or through an open reduction, depending on the site of the fracture, its stability, and/or displacement.

Protection from movement, with casting, splinting, and/or internal fixation to maintain the reduction, is of primary importance to enhance bone healing. *Only* the areas necessary for stabilizing the fracture should be involved in the splint or cast, so that all uninvolved joints and digits can be free to move fully while fracture healing is taking place. Although hand surgeons may differ in their surgical or non-surgical approaches to a specific fracture, they all emphasize the importance of immediate motion of the uninvolved joints and the early mobilization of the joints proximal and distal to the fracture site.[2,4,6-10]

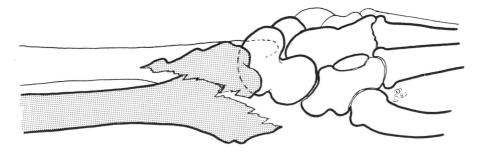

Fig. 10-3.   Barton's fracture: intra-articular fracture with dorsal displacement of the dorsal lip.

Finally, the mobilization of the immobilized areas starts when it is determined that the fracture is "clinically healed." For long bones without internal fixation this usually starts at 3 to 4 weeks post-fracture. When a fracture is fixed internally with K-wires, compression screw, compression plate, or intramedullary rod, motion is usually started immediately. The one exception is the scaphoid or navicular fracture, which is held immobile until there is radiographic evidence that it is healed.[4,7]

WRIST FRACTURES

The three wrist fractures to be discussed, namely the Colles' fracture, the Smith's fracture, and the Barton's fracture, all involve the distal radius. The anatomical location of these fractures, the medical-surgical treatment, the complications, and the therapeutic management of the fractures will be discussed.

The wrist is a frequent site of injury, and the Colles' fracture is probably the most common fracture associated with the wrist (Fig. 10-2).[2,7,11,12] This fracture is at the distal radial shaft, with dorsal or posterior displacement. It can be either extra-articular or intra-articular, and can involve either the distal radio-ulnar joint and/or the radiocarpal joint. Because the usual mechanism of injury is a fall on an outstretched arm, one must not overlook the possibility of a fracture to the radial head or to any of the carpal bones.[2]

Another fracture of the distal radius is Barton's fracture, which is an intra-articular fracture with dorsal displacement of the dorsal lip (Fig. 10-3).[11] Smith's fracture (or reversed Colles' fracture)[2] has a volar displacement of the distal radius giving it a "garden-spade deformity," the opposite of the "dinner-fork deformity" that is seen in Colles' fractures.[11] Smith's fractures are classified into three types. Type I is a transverse fracture through the distal radial shaft. Type II is an oblique fracture through the distal shaft starting at the dorsal articulating lip. Type III (also called a reverse Barton's fracture) is an oblique fracture beginning further down on the articular surface of the radius (Fig. 10-4). The mechanism of injury for these fractures is usually a fall or blow to the dorsum of a flexed hand.[11]

Early Medical Management

Reduction of these fractures is usually closed and sets about to restore proper length, alignment, and articular surfaces. Immobilization in all of these should come distally no further than the mid-palmar crease, in order to allow full flexion and extension of the MCP joints of all the digits.[12]

The position of immobilization of the Colles' fracture is with the wrist in pronation, slight palmar flexion, and about 15 to 20° of ulnar deviation.[12] The cast is placed above the elbow for 2 weeks and is replaced with a short arm cast for another 3 to 4 weeks. Watson-Jones believes that 5 weeks of short arm cast immobilization is long enough to secure union and that there is no need for splinting after this unless there is persistent swelling.[13] Beasley believes that the fracture takes at least 6 to 8 weeks to become secure enough to allow gentle motion at the wrist, and that protective splinting should then be maintained for another 6 to 8 weeks.[4]

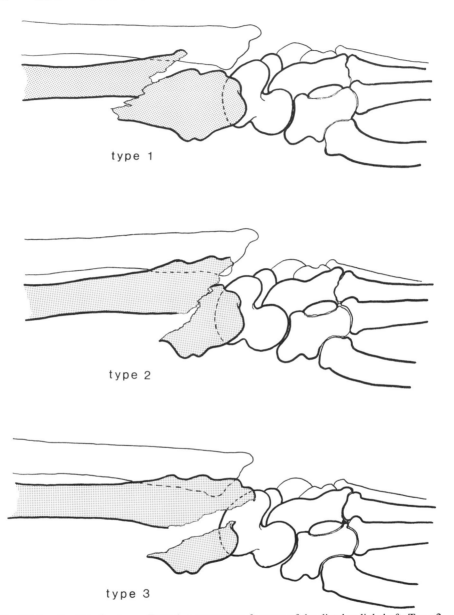

type 1

type 2

type 3

Fig. 10-4.   Smith's fractures: Type 1, a transverse fracture of the distal radial shaft; Type 2, an oblique fracture starting at the dorsal articulating lip; Type 3, an oblique fracture starting further down on the articular surface.

Barton's fractures are less stable, and often displacement occurs. Immobilization is towards the fracture, so a volar fracture is immobilized in slight palmar flexion and a dorsal fracture is set in slight dorsi-flexion.[10] If a large part of the articular surface is disrupted, open reduction and internal fixation are indicated, as the anatomical realignment of the joint surface is important in preventing secondary traumatic joint degeneration.[10]

Smith's fractures are rare, and long arm cast immobilization can be maintained for 5 to 8 weeks, with the wrist in a neutral and supinated position.[11,12] Types II and III tend to be unstable and may require percutaneous K-wire fixation.

Open reduction in wrist fractures is uncommon, and often the end results prove unsatisfactory, considering all the risks involved, but there are cases where it is necessary, such as in realigning the articular surface. If there is a compound fracture with bony loss, such as in a gunshot wound, external fixators may be applied to maintain length during healing.[14]

Hand Therapy

Early Therapeutic Management Immediately Following Closed Reduction. Reduction of edema is of primary importance following any fracture. This is, of course, most simply treated by elevating the hand above the elbow and the elbow above the shoulder.[7] The use of the sling is to be avoided, as this leaves the hand in a dependent position with poor venous drainage. Ice packs can be added in order to decrease the discomfort immediately following the trauma.

Often, swelling is a major factor, causing pain and loss of motion throughout the hand. If that is the case, elevation should be continued, but the use of other modalities will also have to be added. One such modality is the Jobst* intermittent pressure glove, which can be used even if the patient is in a cast, to reduce the swelling in the exposed fingers and thumb. The pressure should be at a point that is well tolerated, not more than 60 to 66 mm Hg pressure. This is usually done for 45 minutes to 1 hour.

Another means of reducing edema is with the use of a Pulse Galvanic Muscle Stimulator, used to activate the muscles around the effected edematous part. The pathological rationale for this treatment is that the muscle pumping action could assist in the absorption process. Alon's monograph cites recent data indicating that acute swelling can also be relieved with electrical stimulation on a sensory excitation level alone, and proposes that there may be an electrical potential field created in the tissues that may trigger the lymphatic system to absorb excessive fluid.[15] This is, as yet, strictly theoretical. When using the Pulse Galvanic Muscle Stimulator, the negative pole is placed over the edematous area, and the positive pole can be placed at some proximal area, usually over the median or ulnar nerve distribution on the upper arm, so that good muscle pump action can be stimulated.[16] Objective circumferential measurements prior to and following treatment will determine the success of the techniques that you are using.

Retrograde milking massage is also helpful in pushing the fluids more proximally, where they can be better absorbed by the body. String wrapping techniques also help in a similar way and can be done to each individual finger, as well as to the exposed metacarpal volar pads. All of these techniques are designed to reduce the swelling so that better active motion can be obtained and maintained by the patient. Wiggling of the fingers does little to reduce fluid, and it does very little to allow excursion of the tendons through the fluid-filled tissue.[4] It is only with strong, forceful, active motion that the excess lymphatic fluid can be expelled from the digits in the hand.[4] These measures

---

*Jobst Inc, Box 653, Toledo, OH 43694.

are temporary, as well, and therefore the swollen hand needs some gentle compressive dressing to maintain the fluid reduction gained in the clinic. Individual digits can be wrapped with coban,* which is an elastic wrap that adheres to itself, or with digital compressive stockinette. The wrap should cover any edematous areas, as wrapping only to the web space will leave the dorsal and volar MP joints as a pocket for fluid moving out of the finger. The patient should be taught how to use these wraps and cautioned about wrapping themselves too tightly, thereby compromising their circulation.

Active and passive range of motion to all uninvolved digits and joints must be started immediately to maintain full range of motion, as well as function. If passive range of motion is needed for any stiff joints, it should be a slow, non-painful form of joint motion, which the patient can continue at home as well as in the clinic. Overzealous patients must be warned that passive range of motion must not be painful, so that they do not inflict any joint trauma upon themselves in their eagerness for improved joint motion.

Active range of motion is aimed at maintaining full joint motion, as well as full tendon excursion of all the muscles involved. Very simply, the major exercises to be done, starting at the most proximal joints and working distally, are (1) full MP flexion, using the lumbricals and interossei, which allows full extension of the PIP and DIP joints, called a lumbrical pull[12]; (2) the individual pull of the sublimis, (3) flexing the PIP joints, coming into a "straight fist" for full sublimis action[16]; (4) full DIP and PIP joint pull using the profundus tendons for the "hook" position; and (5) the use of all three joints being pulled into a full fist, not allowing the thumb to come into adduction.

For the thumb, abduction and IP and MP flexion are started. Abduction and adduction of the fingers are done as well. Any part of the cast not allowing full flexion of the MP joints should be trimmed away. Gradually, active motion is increased with resistance, first using softer objects (such as a nerf ball or half a tennis ball), then the various resistances of theraplast and hand grippers (such as the hand helper† using rubber band resistance).

During this time, full shoulder range of motion exercises and elbow flexion-extension exercises should also be done; incorporating active motion with full flexion of the shoulder up over the head is also an effective means of reducing edema. A note of caution, also: one should check for proper nerve circulation; following fractures to the wrist and excessive edema, median nerve compression at the carpal tunnel could be a problem and would need to be corrected.

Therapeutic Management Following Cast Immobilization. If edema still continues to be a problem, the course of edema control should be continued following cast removal. The various forms of compressive dressings can now involve the wrist and dorsum of the hand, using a compressive type stockinette, the tubigrip glove, or a fabricated Jobst pressure garment. The modalities discussed earlier can also be helpful for edema reduction at the wrist and for regaining range of motion. If you have a patient complying well with the therapy program, that patient should have full range of motion of the thumb and fingers; the primary treatment taking place will be in restoring motion to the wrist. If the fracture is well healed, joint mobilization techniques

---

*3 M Corp, Medical Products Division, St Paul, MN.
†Fred Sammons, Inc, Box 32, Brookfield, IL 60513-0032.

can be very helpful in restoring joint motion following a long period of immobilization. Basically, joint mobilization is a technique to restore normal joint play to a joint.[17] Every synovial joint has a normal joint range of motion, produced by normal muscle action. Besides this normal range of joint motion, there is a subtle but well-defined, small amount of joint play within the joints, which cannot be produced by voluntary muscle activity. It is this joint play that allows easy, painless performance of movements within the voluntary range.[17]

In the wrist there are 16 synovial joints that make up three composite joints. They are the midcarpal joint, the radiocarpal joint, and the ulnomeniscocarpal joint.[17] The normal joint movement of wrist extension takes place at the midcarpal joint, which is made up of the articular surfaces of the scaphoid, the lunate, and the triquetral bones proximally, and the trapezium, trapezoid, capitate, and hamate bones distally. Wrist flexion takes place at the radiocarpal joint, made up of the lower end of the radius and the articulating surfaces of the navicular and the lunate. Supination-pronation is at the ulnomeniscocarpal (ulnomeniscotriquetral) joint and the inferior radio-ulnar joint. The mobilizations that are helpful in regaining extension are at the midcarpal level; they involve long axis extension, anterior-posterior glide, and backward tilt of the distal carpal bones on the proximal row. Mobilizations that increase wrist flexion take place at the radiocarpal joint; they are long axis extension, backward tilt of the navicular and lunate bones on the radius, and the side tilt of the scaphoid on the radius. Supination-pronation can be increased with mobilizations at the ulnomeniscotriquetral joint, using long axis extension, anterior-posterior glide, and the side tilt. At the inferior radioulnar joint, the mobilizations are anterior-posterior glide and the rotation of the lower end of the ulna on the radius. It is important for the therapist to have not only the skill and expertise in the forms of mobilization necessary to increase range of motion, but also the skill in evaluating the source of the pain or the limitation to know that mobilization is in fact the technique necessary to gain the motion needed.[17] For further study on these techniques, I refer you to texts by Mennell,[17] Maitland, and Kaltenborn.

Various heat modalities increasing circulation, decreasing pain, and altering the elasticity of tissues and the viscosity of the synovial joint fluid include warm water soaks, paraffin, and Fluidotherapy.* Although whirlpool is discouraged because the dependent position and the heat add to the swelling, it can be used effectively at 95°C, with active exercises in the water and over the head done alternately throughout the treatment program. Hot packs with elevation can be used. Ice or cryotherapy can be helpful in an extremely painful joint prior to range of motion exercises. Active and passive range of motion exercises to the wrist are started to regain flexion-extension, ulnar and radial deviation, and supination-pronation.

The patient should be instructed in an adequate home therapy program which includes active range of motion exercises at least every 30 to 50 minutes, each particular session lasting 2 to 3 minutes. Pronation and supination exercises should be done with the elbow placed against the wrist at the side to avoid shoulder rotation; these movements appear to involve more pronation or supination then they actually do. If pain is a complicating factor, the use of a transcutaneous nerve stimulator may be helpful during the active range of motion exercises. If relaxation of antagonistic muscles is a problem

---

*Fluido Therapy Corp, 7001 Mullins St, Suite A, Houston, TX 77081.

during active or passive range of motion exercises, the use of biofeedback for relaxation or control of specific muscles may be helpful. The use of an electrical muscle stimulator can increase muscle contraction and aid as an active assistive exerciser. The patient should be instructed that there should be no increase in swelling or pain following any exercise program. The possible reasons for either of these things existing could be too forceful passive range of motion, too long a period of exercise and over straining, or not exercising often enough during the day, thus overworking it when doing exercises.

For patients having open reduction of the wrist, desensitization and friction massage to the scar incision will also be necessary to avoid hypersensitivity, neuroma formation, or adhesion formations blocking full extension or excursion of the tendons. The degree of motion of the wrist expected to return depends upon the age of the person, the severity of the fracture, and the compliance of the patient with the therapy program. Soft tissue tightness, adhesions, and tendon shortening can all be factors affecting the active range of motion. They can be reduced by slow passive range of motion and dynamic splinting. Very little is written as to what exactly constitutes an adequate amount of wrist range of motion; however, in a report by Riggs using the external fixator on 23 patients, the average range of motion following treatment was 48° of wrist flexion, 47° of extension, 26° of ulnar deviation, 11° of radial deviation, 67° of supination, and 62° of pronation.[14] Ten months after treatment, the patient's grip strength was 60 percent of the noninjured hand.

When the fracture is well-healed, the edema is controlled, and joint motion is being regained, strengthening exercises to the wrist need to be started. The flexors can be strengthened with the forearm in a supinated position and the hand extended over the edge of the table or forearm support. The wrist extensors can be strengthened with the forearm pronated and the hand in a flexed position over the table. Radial deviation can be strengthened with the forearm in a midposition and the hand in ulnar deviation, pulling towards a "cocked" or a radial deviated position. Supination-pronation can be strengthened with a one-ended weighted dowel held in the hand and the elbow supported against the body at 90°, moving in both directions.

Daily functional activities and graded work projects can also be used for strengthening, coordination, and endurance prior to returning an injured worker to his job. Strengthening can be done with progressive-resistive exercises, isokenetic equipment or weights made at home. A simple flexion-extension exerciser can be fabricated at home with a pipe or a wooden dowel approximately 2 ft in length, a nylon rope attached at the center, and a 1 or 2 lb weight at the end. The patient standing with the arms extended and the shoulders in 90° of flexion can flex and extend the wrists rolling up the rope or letting it out. These wrist extension exercises are particularly important for any patients who are involved in racquet sports, in order to prevent strain on the extensor tendon, causing a tennis elbow.

Often, regaining wrist range of motion is a very long and arduous process, and knowing when to stop is certainly a question that comes to mind. If the passive range of motion exceeds the active range of motion, weakness of the muscles or adhesions of the tendons are preventing the two from matching. If, at the end range of motion, the resistance feels like a bony block, there may be bony physical limitations that disallow any increased range of motion. If the end ranges of motion feel loose and get painful, more passive followed by active motion may be necessary. If active and passive motion are the same, the patient has good strength, and there has not been an increase in motion for several weeks, one may consider that the maximum range for this particular joint has been reached. Even though the patient may be leaving the clinical setting with an exercise regimen, the patient should be reminded to continue a home program on a regular basis to adequately maintain the gains made. Weakness and loss of motion will ensue if the home program is not continued for several months, or if the patient is not using the hand functionally.

Post-Fracture Complications

The most disabling complication of wrist fractures is the development of reflex sympathetic dystrophy (RSD). A major cause of RSD comes from the painful lesion, associated with swelling at the wrist or direct trauma to the median nerve, called carpal tunnel syndrome. Any complaint of numbness or "deadness" in the fingers, hand, or wrist following a wrist fracture should be heeded as a warning sign of possible nerve problems. Surgical release of the median nerve is done immediately if symptoms exist after a Colles' fracture or crush injuries to the wrist or hand. If no median nerve damage is present, early full active motion reducing the edema in the wrist may prevent this syndrome. If the patient does develop RSD, it takes a tremendous effort on the part of both the patient and the therapist to turn the cycle around and restore function to the hand. Daily therapy for several hours is indicated until the patient's home program is well instituted. A team effort involving the physician, the therapist, the patient and his or her family, and, often, a psychologist or psychiatrist is needed to motivate and encourage the patient to follow through on this rigorous program of therapy needed to restore the mind, body, and hand to a functional level.[2,18]

FRACTURES OF THE DISTAL ULNA

Isolated fractures of the distal ulnar styloid are rare. They are usually caused by a fall onto the ulnar side of an abducted hand. After reduction the site is immobilized in ulnar deviation for 3 to 4 weeks, and for an additional 2 weeks if there is pain or tenderness.

Hand Therapy

The hand therapy for these fractures is essentially the same as that for distal radial fractures. Emphasis may be placed on the return of radial deviation, supination and pronation, and the strengthening of the muscles surrounding this area, namely the flexor carpi ulnaris, extensor carpi ulnaris, and pronator quadratus muscles.

DISLOCATION OF THE DISTAL RADIOULNAR JOINT

This is a common injury, and one often overlooked secondary to other fractures or dislocations of the radius or ulna. The anatomy of this articulation is quite complex, and currently the dysfunction seen clinically is limited. The distal radioulnar joint is stabilized by the triangular fibrocartilage (TFC), which is also known as the carpal articular disc, the triangular ligament, the triangular cartilage or disc, or the meniscus.[19a] The attachment of the TFC to the ulnar head, the lunate, the ulnar styloid process, and the triquetrum as a group is also called the ulnocarpal ligament complex (UCLC).[19a] This is a fibrous system which acts like a hammock extending the gliding surface of the carpals across the width of the forearm, suspending the ulnar aspect of the carpus from the radius and allowing a mechanism of stable rotary movements of the ulnar head while cushioning the forces transmitted through the carpal ulnar axis.[19a] Closely associated with the TFC is a V-shaped ulnocarpal ligament which appears to be one with the TFC in pronation but becomes clearly a separate structure in supination. This combined TFC-UCLC on the ulnar side of the carpus gives it a stabilized rotational attachment to the distal ulna. It is these structures that stabilize the distal radioulnar joint. Bowers states that he found no evidence of a functionally important "ulnar collateral ligament" connecting the carpus to the ulnar styloid.[19a] Please refer to his chapter, The distal radioulnar joint, in *Operative Hand Surgery,* edited by DP Green, MD, for an in-depth look at this anatomically complex joint system.[19a]

Care of the acute intra-articular fracture includes either closed or open reduction, with casting of the wrist in neutral and slight ulnar deviation for 4 weeks. Excision of the ulnar head or replacement of the TFC-UCLC in severely displaced ulnar styloid fractures are fixed with K-wires and require 4 weeks of immobilization in a long arm cast.[19a] With acute joint dislocation in association with other fractures, immobilization is done in a position of mid-rotation, with slight ulnar deviation and volar flexion, the volar ulnar side of the wrist being supported.[19a] Extreme rotation or forced wrist positioning are to be avoided. In isolated dislocations of the distal ulna, 4 to 6 weeks of long arm cast immobilization in pronation is required if the ulna is volarly dislocated, and immobilization is in supination if the ulna is dorsally dislocated.

Delayed Complications of Distal Radioulnar Joint Dislocation

Chronic or late appearing joint derangement (after 2 months) usually has the clinical symptoms of a painful wrist with restricted motion, joint instability, and point tenderness over the articulation. Subluxation may be provoked by full supination, pronation, ulnar deviation, or forceful gripping in any of these positions. Joint surface damage or a discrepancy in the length of the radius or ulna determines which of the many methods will be used to reconstruct this joint. A common one seen for post-traumatic radioulnar joint disease is the Darrach procedure for the operative resection of the distal end of the ulna. Darrach's postoperative management includes no splinting, and active motion is started within 24 hours after surgery.[19a] Complications of this procedure may include ulnar sensory neuroma, radiocarpal rotation, carpal slide, ulnar shaft instability, and rupture of the extensor digiti quinti or extensor digitorum communis.[19a] Immobilization for ulnar head resection can range from 1 week to longer, depending on the amount of bone and soft tissue reconstruction done.

Hand Therapy Following Radioulnar Dislocations

The therapy for radioulnar dislocations when the patient is immobilized in a cast is to maintain reduction of edema and full mobilization and active range of motion of the fingers and thumb. If the dislocation is not immobilized in a cast, but is placed in a protective cock-up splint for 3 to 4 weeks, early active range of motion to the wrist may be ordered by the physician or surgeon. Usually, at 3 weeks following soft tissue arthroplasties, the patient may begin pronation and supination exercises. However, if there is ligament attenuation allowing the ulnar shaft to move dorsally too much during pronation-supination, these exercises may have to be discontinued for a while until the scar tissue is strong enough to hold the radius and ulna in the proper position to allow pain-free pronation-supination. With the surgical management of this kind of injury, the patient must also have scar tissue mobilization to prevent sensory neuromas and adhesions over the extensor carpi ulnaris and extensor digitorium communis. Again, it is very important to build good strength in the wrist, both for the flexors and the extensors, in order to have a pain-free and powerful grasp.

CARPAL FRACTURES/SCAPHOID

Of all wrist injuries, the occurrence of the scaphoid fracture is second in frequency to the fractures of the distal radius and is quite common in young adults.[7,20] The scaphoid may fracture in any of three areas, namely, the middle third or waist, the proximal third, or the distal third, each with a different healing time due to the variance of its blood supply. The mechanism of injury is usually a fall on a dorsiflexed wrist, where the scaphoid is caught between the distal radius and the second carpal row, bending back on the first carpal row.[2,21]

Clinical findings are moderate swelling, pain in the wrist with grasping, and localized tenderness in the anatomical snuffbox and at the scaphoid tubercle.[2,21] If symptoms are present although x-ray is negative, the wrist should be immobilized for 3 weeks and then x-rayed again. Often, these fractures are overlooked because of negative radiographs, but if symptoms are present, they should be treated as fractures. The x-ray will be positive in 3 weeks, when the fracture site will have spread.[7,10,11,21] Because of the vascular supply, these fractures can take up to 6 to 8 months to heal.[4]

Immobilization of Scaphoid Fractures

Fractures of the middle one-third, or waist, of the scaphoid are the most common, and are well known for their high incidence of non-union or delayed union. There is considerable controversy concerning the techniques of immobilization of these fractures. There are three categories of conflict, namely, the wrist position in the cast, the inclusion of other joints such as the elbow or the first three digits, and the length of time in plaster.[21] Since immobilization of the scaphoid is of prime importance to its healing, the cast should be skin-tight so as not to allow any motion at the wrist. Taleisnik believes the thumb to be so intricately related that it should be included in the cast to prevent shearing and compressive forces at the fracture site.[21] Grace in 1929, and Vedan in 1954 suggested inclusion of the elbow to prevent pronation and supination and to eliminate the action of the volar radial carpal ligament on the scaphoid during immobilization.[21] Yet Stewart in 1954 reports on a 95 percent union rate using just a short arm thumb spica cast on a series of 436 fractures.[21] Taleisnik uses the long arm thumb spica for the initial 6 weeks, and then frees the elbow for the remaining time of immobilization.[21] If the fracture shows clinical healing after 8 to 12 weeks, a protective splint may be used which frees the fingers, but still immobilizes the thumb. Conservative treatment with immobilization may continue for 3 to 4 months. If, at that time, the patient is still symptomatic, and there are no signs of fracture healing, a surgical approach would be an alternative.[21]

Fractures of the proximal third of the scaphoid have a high incidence of avascular necrosis or non-union because the vascular supply to the scaphoid is from three vascular systems, all found to be distal to the scaphoid waist.[21] Fractures at this level can take 6 to 11 weeks longer to heal than fractures at the waist or at the middle third.[21] A bone graft, cancellous bone chips, a silastic spacer, or a partial fusion may be used, depending on the size of the bone fragment or the degree of carpal instability.[18,55]

Fractures of the distal third are well vascularized and heal within 3 to 6 weeks. Immobilization is in a short arm thumb spica.

Full active motion of the shoulder, elbow, and noninvolved digits should be encouraged and maintained throughout the course of immobilization. Power grasp is to be avoided while the patient is immobilized, to reduce the chance of stress forces causing movement at the fracture site. Power grasp is not permitted until radiographic evidence of a healed fractured is seen. At this time, full mobilization of the wrist is carried out. Taleisnik believes that range of motion returns rapidly to all uninvolved joints, and full motion should return to the wrist within 1 to 5 weeks following cast removal.[21] Protective splinting may be necessary between exercise periods in the early weeks following cast removal.[4]

CARPAL FRACTURES/TRIQUETRUM

Fractures to the other carpal bones are uncommon, but next in its rate of occurrence is the triquetrum.[21] The mechanism of injury is a fall backward on a dorsiflexed hand forced into ulnar deviation as the patient rolls backward over the ulnar border. Immobilization is for 4 to 6 weeks and causes little, if any, disability.[12,21]

CARPAL FRACTURES/LUNATE

Fractures to the lunate are uncommon but interesting in that if they go undiagnosed or untreated they can result in Keinbock's disease, which will be discussed later. The more common injuries to the lunate are the perilunate dislocation and the lunate dislocation. The difference between them is significant, although Green believes them to be "progressive stages of the same injury"[22] (Fig. 10-5). In a perilunate dislocation, the lunate remains in its normal relationship with the radius, while the proximal carpal row is displaced dorsally to lie on the radius.[22] Mechanism of injury is usually a violent fall from a motorcycle or a height onto an extended hand, which ruptures the posterior ligaments rather than fracturing the distal radius. If the scaphoid is also fractured, this is called a trans-scaphoid perilunate dislocation.

In a lunate dislocation, the bone is exuded through its volar ligaments to lie partially or totally within the carpal tunnel, thus causing compression on the median

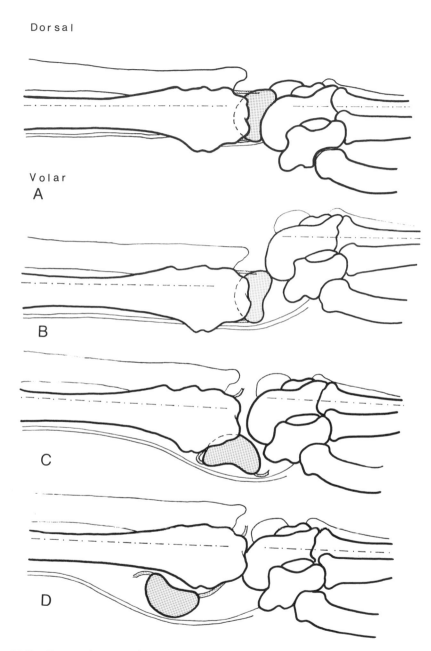

Dorsal

Volar

A

B

C

D

Fig. 10-5. Progressive stages in a lunate dislocation. (A) Normal (B) Perilunate dislocation (C) Position somewhere between the two (D) Lunate dislocation with impingement on the median nerve.

nerve. Its palmar radiocarpal ligament, through which it receives its blood supply, remains attached, so that necrosis of the lunate is not a problem. Clinical symptoms include mild to moderate swelling, diffuse pain about the wrist with limitation in wrist motion, and median nerve paresthesias. Attention should be paid to the neurovascular status of the median nerve, as it may be damaged with the injury.[22] After reduction, immobilization can be anywhere from 5 days to 6 weeks, but during the first 3 weeks the reduction must be reassessed radiographically each week.[22] A short arm thumb spica is then continued for a total of 8 weeks from the time of reduction. There may be significant limitation of motion secondary to articular and ligamentous damage, and a return to heavy labor may take from 6 months to a year.[22]

CARPAL FRACTURES/HAMATE

Fractures of the hamate are either in the body or at the hook. Clinically, there is pain on the ulnar side of the hand, with localized tenderness and swelling over the body of the hamate. These are generally stable fractures and heal with 4 to 6 weeks of immobilization.[21] Symptoms of deep ill-defined pain, that are aggravated by racquet sports or a golf club point to a fracture at the hamular process or hook of the hamate. Recommended treatment is excision of the hook, followed with immobilization until acute tenderness is gone, and then a gradual return to full function.[21]

Hand Therapy

Full, active use of the shoulder, elbow, and non-involved digits should be encouraged and maintained throughout the course of immobilization. Power grasp should be avoided with scaphoid fractures, as any movement during healing could lead to delayed union or non-union. Full mobilization is carried out when radiographic union is seen in any of these carpals. Protective splinting between exercise periods may be necessary in the early weeks following cast removal.

Post-Fracture Complications

The most obvious complication is non-union, which is caused by an insufficient blood supply and/or inadequate immobilization. Treatment for a non-union can be a bone graft,[2,7,21] use of K-wires, screw fixation, proximal row carpectomy,[12,21] or, more recently, a pulsed electrical field in conjunction with bone grafting.[12,23,24] The use of pulsed electromagnetic fields (PEMF) is a noninvasive alternative method for treating non-unions or delayed unions by inducing weak electrical currents into the tissue to modify cell behavior.[23,24] The fibrocartilage calcifies, becomes vascularized, and is then replaced with bone. The main attractions for this treatment seem to lie in its high success rate (84 percent) and its risk-free noninvasive approach.[23,24]

The other major complications involve the lunate and scaphoid bones following fracture. Keinbock's disease is an aseptic necrosis which leads to collapse of the lunate, and Peiser's disease is a similar disorder found in the scaphoid. Although the etiology is not clear, Keinbock's disease appears to be caused by repeated compression of

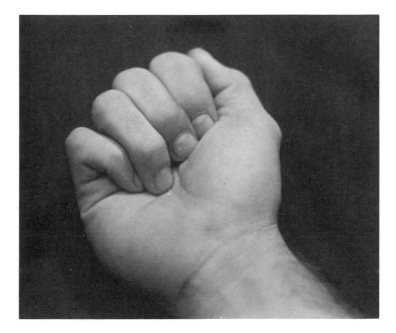

Fig. 10-6. Overlapping of digits in rotational malunion of fifth metacarpal shaft fracture.

the lunate between the radius and capitate, interfering with its healing.[21] Treatment includes lunate implant arthroplasty, intercarpal arthrodesis, wrist arthrodesis, proximal row carpectomy, capitate-hamate fusion, and ulnar lengthening or radial shortening. Rarely is a non-operative method of treatment chosen, as range of motion of the wrist and grip strength gradually decrease.[21]

METACARPAL FRACTURES

Metacarpal features are quite common and can occur at the base, shaft, neck, or head. The mechanism of injury is usually a fall or blow to the fist in a fight. These fractures are usually stable because of the support that they have, with the intrinsic musculature, the interosseous membrane, and their close proximity to their neighboring bones. They have a good blood supply, so they heal quite rapidly and need immobilization for only 2 to 3 weeks, followed by protective splinting for another 2 to 3 weeks.[25] The healing rate will, of course, be faster in the more cancellous bone around the head and base, as compared with a shaft fracture in cortical bone. The distal fragment of a metacarpal fracture will angulate dorsally due to the pull of the interosseous muscles and the flexors.[26] Angulation and rotation are the two major deformities that must be prevented. Rotation at the base, which appears slight, is amplified at the finger tip and can cause an overlapping of the digits in flexion, which is unacceptable (Fig. 10-6). Oblique shaft structures may slide, causing shortening as well as rotation. When a fracture cannot be stabilized with closed reduction or percutaneous K-wires, open reduction and internal fixation with screws, mini plates, or K-wires is used to prevent

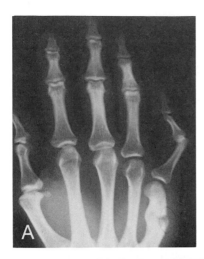

Fig. 10-7. (A) Radiograph of fifth metacarpal fracture with malunion rotational and angulation deformities. (B) Active extension produces hyperextension at the MP joint and an extensor lag at the PIP joint.

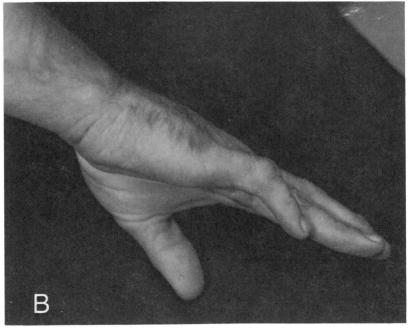

these deformities.[26] Volar angulation is most often seen in a neck fracture of the fourth or fifth metacarpal (boxer's fracture).

Proper immobilization following reduction is imperative to prevent the collateral ligaments, at the metacarpophalangeal joint from retracting and shortening causing an extension contracture. A gutter splint, placing the hand in 70° of flexion at the metacarpophalangeal joint, and extension of the distal joints (clam-digger position), is used for 2 to 3 weeks, after which motion is begun.[25] If volar angulation occurs, it can cause pain when grasping objects, such as a hammer or saw, due to the metacarpal head protruding into the palm.[26] There is differing opinion about what angle is still ac-

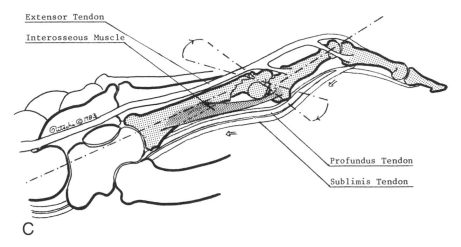

Extensor Tendon

Interosseous Muscle

Profundus Tendon

Sublimis Tendon

C

Fig. 10.7 *(cont.)* (C) Illustration of the zig-zag deformities created by angular malunion.

ceptable without creating a functional deformity. It ranges in fifth metacarpals from 20°[4,26,27] to 70°,[28] as long as there is no rotational deformity. A functional brace for metacarpal fractures has been designed by Betts-Symonds, primarily to free the wrist so the patient can return to work protected at the fracture site, while allowing a greater degree of function.[29]

Using Orthoplast,* a splint is molded around the metacarpals, with pressure molding between them to stretch the interossei, to stabilize the fracture, and to prevent the splint from slipping off. In fifth metacarpal neck fractures, the metacarpophalangeal joint is included, holding it at 90° of flexion.[29]

Hand Therapy

The main goals are to reduce edema, mobilize all uninvolved joints, prevent joint stiffness or contractures, and avoid tendon adherence. The interossei location to the fracture site can cause adhesions and tightening in these muscles and the lateral bands due to inflammation, edema, and direct trauma. The "clam-digger" position also invites intrinsic contracture.[30] Early passive and active flexion of distal and proximal phalangeal joints, while maintaining full extension at the metacarpal joint is necessary to prevent intrinsic contracture.[30] Since the collateral ligaments at the metacarpophalangeal joint are longest in the flexed position, this joint needs attention to prevent an extension contracture. If severe angulation exists at the metacarpal head, the proximal phalanx compensates by assuming a hyperextended, position, extensor lag of the proximal interphalangeal joint results, and a flexion contracture can develop unless prevented (Fig. 10-7). After open reduction, the dorsal incision needs mobilization with friction massage pushing distally against active extension to prevent extensor tendon adhesions.[31] Dorsal swelling is controlled with compression dressings, elevation, pulsed galvanic stimulation, "milking" massage, or Jobst Pump. To control adhesion

---

*Johnson & Johnson

formation, strong, frequent (every 30 minutes), active range of motion exercises are stressed. The importance of the fourth and fifth digits in power grip should not be overlooked in regaining strength and mobility in the hand.

THUMB METACARPAL FRACTURES

First metacarpal fractures can be classified as either extra-articular or intra-articular. Most frequently they occur at the base, but extra-articular fractures of the shaft or near the base cause little or no functional problem with mal-rotation or mal-alignment, due to the compensatory nature of this highly mobile and independent digit. Intra-articular fractures do need precise reduction to minimize joint limitations and prevent secondary arthritic joint changes.[31] The larger the displacement, the more the joint surface is remodeled with fibrocartilage.[2] Residual joint irregularities cause incongruity between the joint surfaces. This inevitably leads to traumatic degenerative joint disease and gradual loss of joint motion or use.[31] In perfectly reduced articular fractures, the thin scar line of fibrocartilage is of little significance.[2]

The two classic intra-articular fractures to the thumb are the Bennett's fracture and the Rolando fracture. Bennett's fracture is between the medial volar lip and the rest of the metacarpal. The volar lip remains attached to the metacarpotrapezial ligament, which prevents subluxation while the metacarpal shaft is pulled radially and dorsally by the abductor pollicis longus.[26] Since Bennett first described this fracture in 1882, there have been 19 different treatments advocated, all reporting good results.[26] The most recent trend is toward an ASIF cancellous screw, which allows precise alignment of the articular surfaces while affording the stability for immediate mobilization.[26] When the fracture is reduced with percutaneous K-wires, the patient is placed in a thumb spica for 4 weeks, after which motion is started.[26] The pins are removed after 6 weeks.

Another method of immobilization for Bennett's fractures, which allows wrist motion was developed by Betts-Symond. After reduction, the thumb is splinted in abduction from the base to include the interphalangeal joint. A separate forearm cuff is made with a hinge at the wrist attaching the thumb splint, allowing only wrist flexion and extension, as ulnar deviation displaces the fracture laterally. Fracture bracing is becoming more popular, as it allows the limb to function in as normal a way as possible while immobilizing the fracture.

A Rolando fracture is Y-shaped, with both a volar and a dorsal fragment. These can be fixed with K-wires, a small buttress plate, or, if severely comminuted, molded in plaster with the metacarpal in palmar abduction for 3 to 4 weeks.[26]

Another common thumb injury is the acute rupture of the ulnar collateral ligament of the metacarpophalangeal joint. This injury is inaccurately referred to as gamekeeper's thumb, which is really a chronic stretch injury.[4] The most common mechanism of injury is a fall on an abducted thumb, seen in a high percentage of skiing injuries.[32] If total separation exists between the ulnar collateral ligament and the base of the first phalanx, the adductor tendon can interpose between the ligament and its normal position, in which case surgery is indicated to prevent loss of pinch. Immobilization is in a thumb spica with slight ulnar deviation at the metacarpophalangeal joint for 6 weeks.

Hand Therapy

Since the thumb is considered to be 60 percent of the hand, regaining its mobility, coordination, and strength are the main objectives of therapy. Having to immobilize any joint for 3 to 6 weeks leaves it tight, stiff, and weak. Joint mobilization and dynamic flexion splinting, as well as passive and active range of motion exercises are needed to regain motion, flexibility, coordination, and pinch strength. The habit of using the index and middle fingers for pinch, excluding the thumb, may be altered by placing a buddy splint on them, disallowing the index finger opposition and abduction to the middle finger. Scar mobilization over the dorsal incision helps remodel the scar connected to the extensor pollicis longus tendon that may have formed. Full use is restricted for 3 to 4 months after collateral ligament repair.[33]

Complications

Complications include malunion, which may allow recurrent subluxation of the metacarpotrapezial joint or poor joint surface alignment, causing secondary arthritis and pain. Both can be corrected with arthrodesis of the carpometacarpal joint. A complication to the ulnar collateral ligament injury ligament attenuation caused by early excessive motion of the thumb, leading to joint instability and loss of pinch power and/or symptoms of pain. Arthrodesis of the metacarpophalangeal joint will correct this problem.

PHALANGEAL FRACTURES

Phalangeal fractures are the most common fractures in the hand and are often the most complicated. Because the tendons and neurovascular bundles are in such close proximity to the bones, soft tissue injury as well as the fracture results. Edema, joint stiffness, tendon adhesions, hypersensitivity, and fearful patients are but a few of the obstacles to be overcome.

DISTAL PHALANGEAL FRACTURES/INTRA-ARTICULAR

Commonly, an intra-articular fracture of the distal phalanx is called a mallet or baseball finger. This name has been applied to two different types of fractures, and the distinction between the two is important, as it affects both the treatment and the prognosis.[34] A true mallet finger with a fracture involves the avulsion of the extensor tendon; the other is a dorsal fracture at the distal phalangeal base with no associated tendon rupture.[34] The latter involves a volar subluxation of the terminal phalanx producing swelling over the distal joint, thus appearing to be a tendon avulsion or mallet finger.[34] In spite of the fracture, the extensor expansion does not lose its attachment to the distal phalanx, so no drooping occurs. The injury is usually caused by a blow to the end of the finger causing a longitudinal compression and hyperextension of the distal

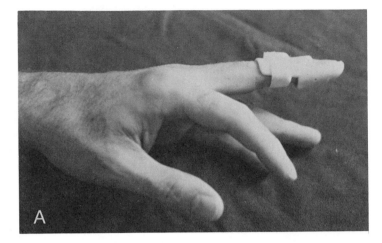

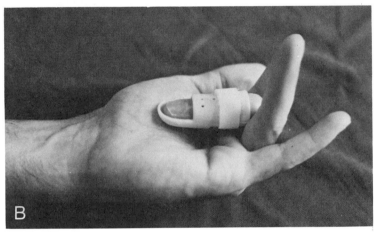

Fig. 10-8. (A) Mallet finger with Stack Splint holding distal joint in extension, (B) while allowing full flexion at the proximal joints.

phalanx.[34] Because the tendon is still intact, early motion can be started with splinting done for comfort.[34] If a large articular fragment is present with volar subluxation, the distal joint is splinted in flexion for adequate reduction. If lateral x-rays show this does not reduce the fracture adequately, internal fixation may be used.[34]

In the distal phalangeal fracture with mallet finger, the extensor tendon is avulsed from the distal phalanx, and the immobilization following reduction can be done with external splinting (Fig. 10-8) (Slack splint* or Orthoplast-type) or K-wires, placing the phalanx in slight hyperextension, (Fig. 10-9). A study comparing internal versus external splintage showed no difference in terms of results between the two forms, but did find that early treatment was a factor for success.[35] Immobilization is for 6 weeks, allowing and encouraging PIP and MP joint motion.[35]

---

*Link America, 10 Great Meadow Lane, E. Hanover, NJ 07936.

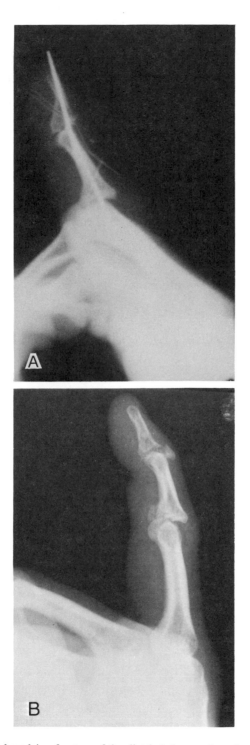

Fig. 10-9. (A) Dorsal avulsion fracture of the distal phalanx and a volar intra-articular fracture subluxation involving 55 percent of the articular surface of the PIP joint. (B) X-ray showing use of a K-wire and intra-osseous wire fixation with pull-out suture for the tendon repair.

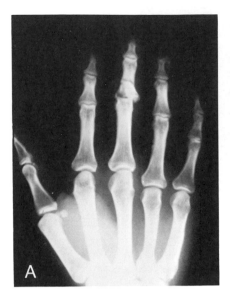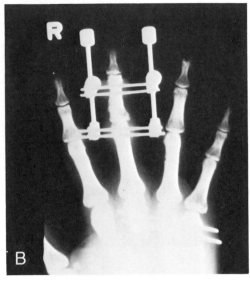

Fig. 10-10.   (A) Severely comminuted T-type fracture at the base of the middle phalanx with subluxation; oblique mid-shaft fracture in the metacarpal with distal tuft fracture in the middle finger. (B) Matev distraction device used as external fixature to maintain length.

Hand Therapy

Therapy to the distal joint is started following splint or K-wire removal at approximately 6 weeks.[35] Isolated flexion-extension exercises can be done by blocking the proximal joints. A careful balance is needed in regaining flexion to the joint without losing active extension by tendon attenuation.[25] This can be prevented by static splinting either between exercise periods or at nighttime for an additional 2 weeks. Belsole believes that a proximal shift in the length of the digital extensor tendon alters the coordination of motion in the phalanges thus compromising hand function.[27] In many cases of distal fractures, treated or untreated, there may be a residual loss of active extension.[36]

MIDDLE PHALANGEAL
FRACTURES/EXTRA-ARTICULAR

Extra-articular fractures can occur at any level of the middle phalanx, but their displacement will vary depending on the level of the fracture.[1] Fractures in the distal one-fourth displace or angulate volarly due to the pull of the sublimis tendon. Fractures in the middle two-fourths can angulate in either direction and are unstable, often needing internal fixation.[1] Fractures in the proximal one-fourth will angulate dorsally due to the un-balanced pull of the extensor tendon (Flatt) or the pull of the sublimis tendon on the distal fragment (McNealy and Lichtenstein).[1] Transverse fractures of the middle

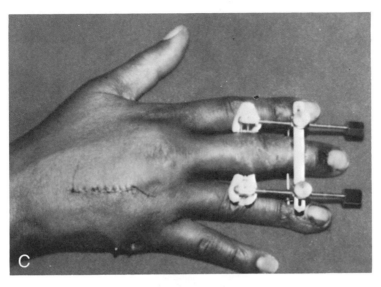

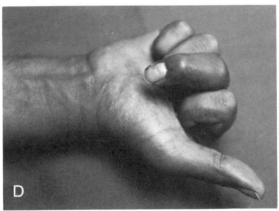

Fig. 10.10 (*cont.*)   (C) External fixation allows for active motion of joints distal and proximal to fracture site. (D) Active flexion by patient 10 weeks post-fracture and 6 weeks after removal of the device.

phalangeal shaft take longer to heal (10 to 14 weeks) due to the large amount of cortical bone involved.[1,21] Displaced phalangeal fractures need early mobilization to prevent joint stiffness and allow tendon gliding. Rigid stabilization and early motion follow as the best means of obtaining these functional goals. Because of the difficulty in obtaining a good reduction with closed pin fixation, open reduction using K-wires, compression or tension bands, mini-screws, or a combination of interosseous wire and K-wires (Fig. 10-10) may be used.[37] Compression plates are not advocated for use in the phalanges because of the extensive tissue disruption involved in placing them.[27] With severe comminution, an external fixature (Matev, mini-Hoffman) can be used to maintain length and prevent rotation, while active motion to the other joints, proximal and distal to the fracture is encouraged. Traction is rarely used because of the complications associated with its application, counter-pressure forces involved, and the resultant joint stiffness.[1]

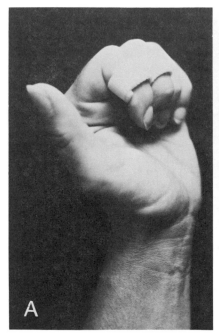
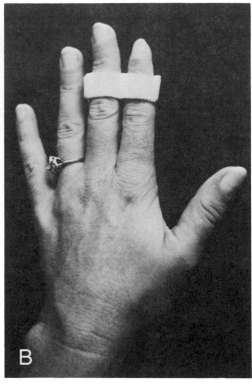

Fig. 10-11. (A) Buddy splint to protect non-displaced fracture of middle phalanx of the index finger, allowing flexion, and (B) extension while giving lateral support.

Hand Therapy

The primary concern in treating middle phalangeal fractures is regaining and maintaining full motion at the joints proximal and distal to the fracture site. With displaced comminuted or intra-articular fractures, the likelihood of flexor tendon or extensor tendon damage is quite good, and adherence to the bony callus creates contractures and limits active and passive range of motion. Prevention of these contractures and restoring tendon glide over the healing fracture is vital. Obviously, early mobilization (after 5 to 15 days) with good fracture stabilization is the best way to treat these fractures. Stabilizing the phalanx just proximal to the joint being exercised gives good support for individual joint range of motion.[10,31] Strapping the digit to the adjacent finger (Buddy splinting) is both a dynamic splint, allowing active and active-assistive motion, and a protective splint, giving lateral support. (Fig. 10-11) Immobilization of the DIP joint should not exceed 3 weeks, as this can cause residual joint stiffness. When PIP joint immobilization is necessary, it should be done in extension (0 to 10°) to prevent a flexion contracture.[27] If the extensor tendon has been cut to allow placement of a fixation device, the distal interphalangeal joint is protected from active flexion. By developing the sublimis tendon, proximal interphalangeal joint motion is maintained until distal motion is started at 3 weeks. Since normal flexor tone pulls the phalanges into flexion, it is probable that without intervention the proximal interphalangeal joint will

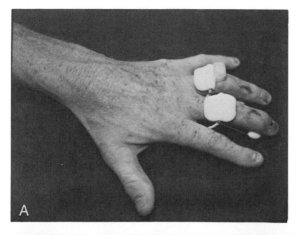

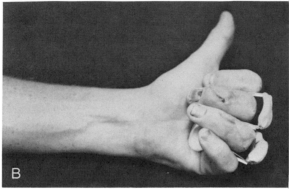

Fig. 10-12. Fractures to third and fourth middle phalanges with K-wire fixation. (A) In dynamic extension splints to prevent joint contracture (note dorsal bar has been cut away to take pressure off the protruding K-wire). (B) Splints give gentle resistance during active flexion.

develop a flexion contracture. A nighttime splint holding the PIP joint in neutral will override this natural pull, preventing a shortening of the soft tissue structures surrounding this joint. When the fracture is stable, alternating dynamic flexion with dynamic extension splinting can be helpful in restoring motion. The LMB* active extension splint and the Capner† splint are good for individual joint extension, but caution should be taken to watch for dorsal swelling just proximal to the dorsal stabilizer (Fig. 10-12).

MIDDLE PHALANGEAL FRACTURES WITH VOLAR PLATE INVOLVEMENT

A common complication to a hyperextension injury of the finger is rupture of the volar plate, the anterior stabilizing structure of the proximal interphalangeal joint. When the rupture occurs at its distal attachment, a fragment of bone may be avulsed

---

*LMB Hand Rehab Products, 111 Nieto Ave, Long Beach, CA 90803.
†Roylan Manufacturing Co, Inc, PO Box 555, Menomonee Falls, WI 53051.

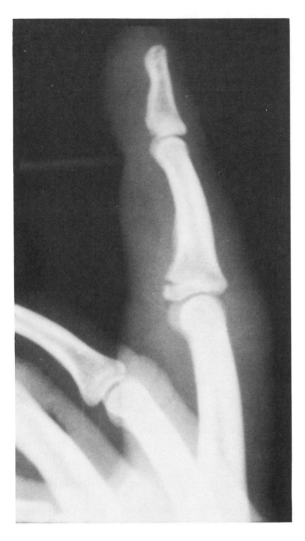

Fig. 10-13.   Radiograph of volar plate fracture.

from the base of the middle phalanx.[33,37,38] Diagnosis is made by clinical findings of anterior proximal interphalangeal joint pain or tenderness, pain with hyperextension, and instability with loss of pinch power.[38] With careful attention to cortical detail, the chip or fragment can be seen on a lateral or oblique view radiographically[38] (Fig. 10-13). Frequently these injuries are associated with sports. Hence, they are more common in young adults, and their incidence is greater in the fall and early spring.[38]

Treatment, if the fragment is undisplaced, is immobilization in 30° of flexion for 2 weeks, followed by active exercises in a dorsal block splint preventing extension at 15°[4,33] (Fig. 10-14). Full extension is allowed after 6 weeks. Open reduction with internal fixation is indicated if more than 30 percent of the articular surface is involved.[33] Careful and accurate reduction of the articular surface is necessary to prevent permanent joint stiffness and secondary arthritis. The PIP joint needs to be placed in flexion for adequate reduction and is pinned in 30° of flexion for 10 days to 14 days.[27]

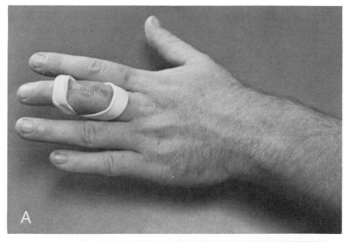

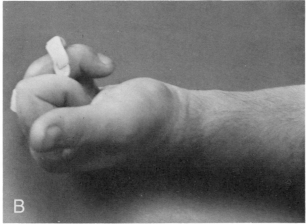

Fig. 10-14. (A) Dorsal extension block splint limiting extension at 15 degrees and (B) allowing full flexion of the joints.

Hand Therapy

Care is again taken to reduce edema and begin active motion to all joints not involved. During the immobilization period, the metacarpophalangeal and distal phalangeal joints must be kept moving to prevent stiffness and adhesions, especially at the bifurcation of the sublimis to the profundus tendon. When the K-wire is removed at 2 weeks, active flexion-extension exercises are started using a dorsal block splint to prevent the final degrees of extension. Splinting is maintained for 2 more weeks, and full active extension is started at 4 weeks post-surgery.[27] Dynamic extension splinting is started at 5 weeks, if full active extension has not been regained.[33] Belsole believes a dynamic dorsal extension splint is most often necessary to achieve and maintain full PIP joint extension.[27] It may take 6 to 8 months after the injury for PIP joints to fully loosen and for the swelling to subside.[4,39] Educating the patient in the severity of this injury and its long course to recovery may save him/her some frustration as he/she struggles to regain a functional and pain-free joint.[33] Failure to treat the volar plate rupture can lead to late complications, including recurrent subluxation, flexion contracture, hyperextension of the PIP joint due to relaxation in the extensor mechanism (Swan neck deformity), and traumatic arthritis.[38]

PROXIMAL PHALANGEAL FRACTURES

There are several reasons why proximal phalangeal fractures are of such concern to us. Of all phalangeal fractures, they occur twice as often as middle or distal phalangeal fractures.[7] They are the structural center between the two most important joints in the hand, and they invariably involve the surrounding soft tissue, namely the flexor and extensor tendons and the neurovascular bundles. Malalignment in either rotation or angulation can cause significant dysfunction in the hand. Rotational deformities cause overlapping of the adjacent digit in flexion, while angulation causes contracture due to the muscle imbalance. The fractures can occur at any level and all have inherent problems associated with them. The proximal or base fractures involve the flexor tendon sheath and/or the metacarpophalangeal joint; distal head or neck fractures involve the proximal interphalangeal joint; and the mid-shaft fractures are often unstable spiral or oblique breaks leading to shortening or rotational deformities. Healing time for most proximal phalangeal fractures is 5 to 7 weeks for clinical union with complete radiographic bone healing seen at about 5 months.[26] Extra-articular nondisplaced phalangeal fractures are usually stable due to their relatively intact periosteal tube.[2] Treatment is Buddy splinting with immediate motion.[2,7,8,25,26]

Displaced fractures can be reduced with either a closed or an open method. When casting these fractures, the metacarpophalangeal joint is in flexion (70°) and the proximal interphalangeal joint is in extension (clam-digger position).[25,27] Open reduction with internal fixation can include K-wire, intraosseous wiring, compression screws, or an intra-medullary rod.[27] Fractures in the proximal or distal third involve more cancellous bone and therefore rapidly heal in about 3 weeks. The middle third is mainly cortical bone needing 4 to 6 weeks of immobilization to allow healing and protection from displacement.

Intra-articular fractures need a stable, congruous joint surface to restore satisfactory motion and a stable, painless joint. Nondisplaced articular fractures are anatomically stable with minimal joint disruption, so immobilization is only needed for 2 to 3 weeks before active exercise is initiated. Displaced articular fractures need open reduction to accurately realign the joint surface and prevent secondary joint degeneration. Indications for open reduction in these fractures are instability, incongruity, irreducibility, and interposition of soft tissue. K-wire fixation is held for at least 6 weeks in these intra-articular fractures, since their healing is somewhat delayed.[26]

Hand Therapy

Stiffness is the major problem in phalangeal fractures, and prevention is far better than the cure. Prolonged immobilization and extensive soft tissue swelling are the two major causes of fibrosis and ankylosing of the joints. Early mobilization is initiated (at

5 to 15 days) when internal fixation is providing stability at the fracture site.[25] When a cast or splint is used, only the joints distal and proximal to the fracture, (and if necessary the adjacent digit), are immobilized, and all other joints are kept moving. Edema is controlled with elevation, compressive dressing (Coban, Compresso-grip)*, and modalities such as Jobst Pump or pulsed galvanic muscle stimulation. When the fracture is stable, dynamic and/or static splinting may be necessary to prevent or correct a contracture, or to aid in gaining passive joint motion. Tendon adhesions can be avoided with early, continuous active exercises aimed at full tendon excursion in both directions.[24] Friction massage is used to mobilize the scar and to free tendon and nerve adhesions. By applying deep friction in a distal direction as the patient actively extends his joint, adhesions to the extensor tendon can be stressed.[31] Electrical muscle stimulators (Faradic current) or biofeedback techniques can enhance muscle contraction, thus aiding joint and tendon movements.

The most important thing is to stress, encourage, cajole, or bribe the patient into full motion to limit the complications inherent with the "waiting-for-the-pain-to-go-away-first" attitude. Joint range of motion exercises need to be done for 2 to 3 minutes every half hour. Exercises done only three to five times a day are not adequate to offset the joint stiffness associated with phalangeal fractures. Strengthening begins when a fracture is "clinically" united and progresses as long as there is no pain at the fracture site. Fractures can refracture even after 8 weeks, if the stress placed on them is too great.[40] Joint stiffness, joint swelling, cold intolerance, and pain on extremes of motion may continue for up to a year after phalangeal fractures. A study reviewing the functional results of patients with metacarpal or phalangeal fractures was done by Weeks and Wray showing that the best total active motion (average $TAM = 200°$) was achieved by patients with a single phalangeal or metacarpal fracture. Patients with more than one fracture per hand or a fracture to the proximal phalanx had less active motion (average $TAM = 174°$). Crush injuries with multiple fractures or more than one fracture per finger had the least amount of active motion recovery (average $TAM = 130°$)[31,41] Significant differences in passive ROM versus active ROM in all cases showed the patient to be unable to achieve the full active potential due to adhesions along the musculotendonous unit.[31]

Complications

Complications include: mal-rotation (as little as 10 percent can cause digital overlapping); malunion with angulation; non-union (more often it is delayed union); and loss of motion due to either tendon adhesions or joint contracture. Extensor tendon adherence will limit proximal interphalangeal joint flexion actively and passively, and will limit active extension but not passive extension. Adhesions of the sublimus tendon cause limited active and passive extension of the proximal interphalangeal joint, while full flexion is achieved by the profundus tendon. Surgical intervention to correct both joint contracture and tendon adhesions is difficult and often yields only slight improvement. Rupture of the flexor tendon following screw fixation and percutaneous pinning has been seen.[3,26]

---

*All Orthopedic Appliances, 74 N.E. 75th St., Miami, Fl. 33138

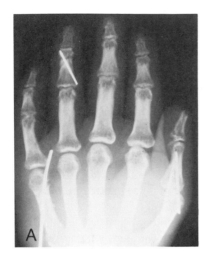
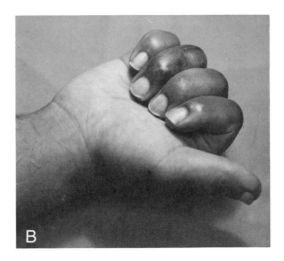

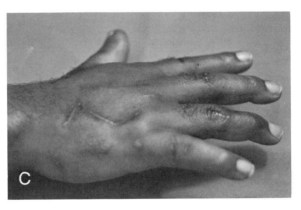

Fig. 10-15. A 26-year-old male sustained multiple fractures and soft tissue damage when a 1200 pound safe landed on his right hand. (A) Open reduction with K-wire fixation to the fractures of his fifth metacarpal, the middle phalanx of his ring finger, the proximal phalanx of his thumb, and amputation of the tip of his thumb. (B) After early motion (6 days) his flexion at 8 weeks post-op, and (C) His extension at 8 weeks post-op.

MULTIPLE FRACTURES OR BONY LOSS

Multiple fractures or severe bony loss (gunshot wounds) are usually caused by direct violence to the hand. With these, extensive soft tissue damage is seen and the rate of fracture healing is slower due to the vascular damage. These fractures are generally treated with open reduction and debridement; in compound fractures with primary or secondary wound closure, internal fixation, and early motion (Fig. 10-15). Complicating factors are severe or persistant edema and/or infection, both of which lead to joint stiffness. Rigid skeletal fixation is useful in preventing or dealing with bone infection, and it also allows early motion. An aggressive approach is needed in working with multiple fractures to maintain joint motion and prevent adhesions. Treating the soft tissue injury as primary and more or less ignoring the fractures may be a more valuable way of approaching treatment of these horrendous injuries.

Hand Therapy

All the complications facing the single fracture are multiplied in the severely injured hand. A dynamic approach is needed to address all the problems in a systematic way. Firstly, educating the patient for compliance with the home program and assuming the major active role in his rehabilitation process should be started immediately and reinforced throughout his course of treatment. Using the various techniques and modalities outlined earlier, the priorities of care are: proper and adequate skeletal fixation to support healing bone tissue, wound care to open wounds for optimal healing with minimal scar formation, edema control to minimize fibrosis and joint stiffness, full active tendon excursion to prevent adhesions, pain control as needed, joint mobilization to regain any lost joint play and range of motion, and splinting as needed to prevent joint contractures. Modalities of heat, cold, electrical stimulation, or biofeedback are added to the treatment as needed. Objective measurements are taken to assess the effectiveness of the treatment and to evaluate the progress of the patient. As healing progresses, desensitization, progressive resistive exercise, and functional activities are incorporated into the therapy program.

SUMMARY

Fractures of the wrist and hand are common injuries which are often underrated with little appreciation given to the associated soft tissue damage. When mismanaged or left untreated, significant functional impairment may occur. These complications can be minimized by a dynamic and thorough approach following the basic tenets outlined for fracture healing. Patient education, proper immobilization, and early protected motion to decrease joint stiffness and enhance tendon gliding are of primary importance for a good end result.

ACKNOWLEDGEMENT

I gratefully acknowledge the grant I received from the National Hand Research and Rehabilitation Fund.

REFERENCES

1. McKibbin B: The biology of fracture healing in long bones. J Bone Joint Surg 60:150, 1978
2. Salter RB: Textbook of Disorders and Injuries of the Musculoskeletal System. Williams & Wilkins Co, Baltimore, 1970
3. Elkouri ER: Review of cancellous and cortical bone healing after fracture or osteotomy. J Am Podiatr Assoc 72:464m 1982

4. Beasley RW: Hand Injuries. WB Saunders Co, Philadelphia, 1981
5. Alexander H et al: Development of new methods for phalangeal fracture fixation. J Biomech 14:377, 1981
6. Barton NJ: Fractures of the shafts of the phalanges of the hand. The Hand 11:119, 1979
7. Boyes JH: Bunnell's Surgery of the Hand. JB Lippincott Co, Philadelphia, 1964
8. Clinkscales GS: Displaced and nondisplaced fractures in the hand. In Cowen NJ (ed): Practical Hand Surgery. Symposia Specialists, Chicago, 1980
9. Imbriglia JE: Articular fractures and fracture dislocations. In Cowen NJ (ed): Practical Hand Surgery. Symposia Specialists Inc, Chicago, 1980
10. Wilson RL, Carter MS: Management of hand fractures. In: Rehabilitation of the Hand, Hunter JM, Schneider LH, Mackin EJ, Bell JA (eds) CV Mosby Co, St. Louis, 1978
11. Conwell HE: Injuries to the Wrist. In Walton JH (ed): Clinical Symposia. Ciba, New Jersey, 1970
12. Frykman GK, Nelson EF: Fractures and traumatic conditions of the wrist. In Hunter JM, Schneider LH, Mackin EJ, Callahan AD (eds): Rehabilitation of the Hand-2nd Edition, CV Mosby Co, St Louis, 1984
13. Watson-Jones R: Fractures and Joint Injuries. Williams & Wilkins Co, Baltimore, 1944
14. Riggs SA, Conney WP: External fixation of complex hand and wrist fractures. J Trauma 23:332, 1982
15. Alon G: High Voltage Galvanic Stimulation. A monograph.
16. Sorenson MK: Pulsed galvanic muscle stimulation for post-op edema in the hand. Pain Control, Number 37, 1983
17. Mennell JMcM: Joint Pain. Little, Brown and Co, Boston, 1964
18. Lankford LL: Reflex sympathetic dystrophy. In Green DP (ed): Operative Hand Surgery. Churchill Livingstone, New York, 1982
19. Bowers WH: Capsular injuries of the proximal interphalangeal joint. In Cowen NJ (ed): Practical Hand Surgery. Symposia Specialists, Inc, Chicago, 1980
19a. Bowers WH: Distal radioulnar joint. In Green DP (ed): Operative Hand Surgery. Churchill Livingstone, New York, 1982
20. Harris WH, Jones WN, Aufranc OE: Fracture Problems. CV Mosby Co, St Louis, 1965
21. Taleisnik J: Fractures of the carpal bones. In Green DP (ed): Operative Hand Surgery. Churchill Livingstone, New York, 1982
22. Green DP: Carpal dislocations. In Green DP (ed): Operative Hand Surgery. Churchill Livingstone, New York, 1982
23. Bassett CAL et al: Pulsing electromagnetic field treatment in ununited fractures and failed arthrodeses. JAMA, 247:623, 1982
24. Bassett CAL, Mitchell SN, Schink MM: Treatment of therapeutically resistant non-unions with bone grafts and pulsing electromagnetic fields. J Bone Joint Surg 64:1214, 1982
25. Wilson RL, Carter MS: Management of hand fractures. In Hunter JM, Schneider LH, Mackin EJ, Callahan AD (eds): Rehabilitation of the Hand, 2nd Edition, CV Mosby Co, St Louis, 1984
26. O'Brien ET: Fractures of the metacarpals and phalanges. In Green DP (ed): Operative Hand Surgery. Churchill Livingstone, New York, 1982
27. Belsole R: Physiological fixation of displaced and unstable fractures. Orthop Clin North Am 11:393, 1980
28. Hunter JM, Cowen NJ: Fifth metacarpal fractures in a compensation clinic population. J Bone Joint Surg 52-A:1159, 1970
29. Betts-Symonds GW, Bell AP: Functional bracing of metacarpal fractures. Nurs Times Nov: 1995, 1982

30. Wilson RL, Carter MS: Joint injuries in the hand & preservation of proximal interphalangeal joint function. In Hunter JM, Schneider LH, Mackin EJ, Bell JA (eds): Rehabilitation of the Hand, CV Mosby Co, St Louis, 1978

31. Weeks PM, Wray RD: Management of Acute Hand Injuries, A Biological Approach. CV Mosby Co, St Louis, 1978

32. Carr D, Johnson RJ, Pope MH: Upper extremity injuries in skiing. Am J Sports Med 9:378, 1981

33. Eaton RG, Dray GJ: Dislocations and ligament injuries in the digit. In Green DP (ed): Operative Hand Surgery, Churchill Livingstone, New York, 1982

34. McMinn DJW: Mallet finger and fractures. Injury. The British Journal of Accident Surgery 12:477, 1981

35. Auchincloss JM: Mallet finger injuries: A prospective, controlled trial of internal and external splintage. The Hand 14:168, 1982

36. Barton NJ: Fractures of the phalanges of the hand. The Hand 9:1, 1977

37. Baugher WH, McCue FC: Anterior fracture-dislocation of the proximal interphalangeal joint. J Bone Joint Surg 61-A:799, 1979

38. Nance EP, Kaye JJ, Milek MA: Volar plate fractures. Radiology 133:61, 1979

39. Eaton RG, Malerich MM: Volar plate arthroplasty of the proximal interphalangeal joint: A review of ten year's experience. J Hand Surg 5:260, 1980

40. Whiteside J, Fleagle S, Kalevak A: Fractures and refractures in intercollegiate athletes. Am J Sports Med 9:369, 1981

41. Huffaker WH, Wray RC, Weeks PM: Factures influencing final range of motion in the fingers after fractures of the hand. Plast Reconstr Surg 63:82, 1979

Index

Page numbers followed by f represent figures; page numbers followed by t represent tables.

Adhesion formation, and replantation therapy, 113-115
ADL intervention, in replantation therapy, 99-100
Alumafoam technique, splinting, 178-179, 180f
Amputations. *See* Replantation
Anatomy
  arches, 161-162, 162f
  flexion creases, 164-165, 164f
  hand/upper extremity functional unit, 160-161
  ligamentous, 163-164
  muscular, 162-163
  osseous, 161
  and vasomotor disabilities, 72-73
Anoxia, and replantation therapy, 92
Anti-boutonniere splint, 173, 176f
Anti-Swan neck splint, 173, 174f-175f
Anxiety, and pain perception, 148
Arches, anatomy, 161-162, 162f
Arthroplasty, 117-134
  carpometacarpal joint arthroplasty, 122-123
  first generation implants
    long-term follow-up, 123-124
    postoperative management, 124-125
  the future, 132
  generations of implants, 119-122
  historical perspective, 117-118
  long-term results, 130-132
    function issues, 131
    infection and, 131-132
    patient satisfaction, 132
    prosthetic fracture and, 131
    range of motion, 132
  postoperative care, 127-130
    clinical studies, 129
    metacarpophalangeal, 127
    proximal interphalangeal joint, 128-129
    third generation implants, 130
    variables affecting, 127-130

second generation implants, 125-127
  axes of rotation, 126-127
  surgery candidates, 126
Avascular zones, in digital flexor tendon, 20f
Avulsion injury. *See* Replantation

Barton's fracture, 195-201, 196f
Bennett's fracture, 210
Biofeedback, 11, 109
Biomechanical principles, of splinting, 167-168
  forces, 168
  levers, 167
  pressure, 168
  three point pressure system, 168
Blood supply
  of flexor tendon, 19, 19f
  and tendon repair, 27
Bony loss, 222-223
Boutonniere deformity, 129
Braille designs, and sensory re-education, 62
BTE Work Simulator, 139
Buddy straps, 104
Buddy system splint, 182-183, 186f, 216f

Capener splints, 104, 183, 187f, 217
Capsulotomies, and pain management, 150
Carpal fractures, 203-207
  hamate, 206-207
  lunate, 204-206, 205f
  scaphoid, 203-204
  triquetrum, 204
Carpal tunnel syndrome, 152, 154
Carpectomy, proximal row, 206
Carpometacarpal joint arthroplasty, 122-123, 122t
  complications, 123, 124t
  indications, 122

Carpometacarpal joint arthroplasty (*cont.*)
   postoperative management, 122
   postoperative results, 123
Coban wrappings, 100, 152, 153f
Cold intolerance, and replantation, 115
Collagen production, and wound remodelling,
   7-8
Colles' fracture, 195-201, 194f
Contact inhibition, 6
Contracture, joint, 6
Crush injury. *See* Replantation

Darrach procedure, 202
De Quervains' syndrome, 154-155, 155f
Diathesis, 156
Dictionary of Occupational Titles, 141
Discrimination training, and sensory re-educa-
   tion, 59
Distal interphalangeal joint injuries, 35-36
   immobilization period, 35-36
   mobilization period, 36
Distal ulna fracture, 201
Dynamic splinting, 166-167. *See also*
   Splinting
   custom fabricated, 179-183
   commercially fabricated, 183
   thumb splints, 183, 186f

Edema, and wound healing, 3-4, 4f
Elastomer inserts, 103
Electrical stimulation, and tendon gliding, 11
Extensor habitus, 152, 152f
Extensor hood injuries, 33-35
   anatomical considerations, 33, 33f
   immobilization period, 34
   mobilization period, 34-35
   proximal interphalangeal joint level, 33-34
Extensor tendon injuries, common, 29-33
   anatomical considerations, 29-30
   immobilization period and techniques, 30
   mobilization period and techniques, 30-31
   new approaches, 31-33
   splinting, 32f
Extensor tendon management, 27-36. *See also*
   Tendon healing
   by level of injury, 29-36
      common extensor, 29-33
      distal interphalangeal joint, 35-36
      extensor hood, 33-35
      general considerations, 27-29
Extrinsic healing, tendon, 22-23, 24, 22f

Fabrication, splint, 170-173. *See also*
   Splinting
Fibroplasia phase, of wound healing, 5-6
Finger mazes, and sensory re-education, 62,
   62f
Finger trapper splint, 182-183, 186f
Finkelstein test, 154, 155f
Flatt prosthesis, 120f
Flexion creases, 164-165
   digital, 164-165
   palmar, 165
   wrist, 165
Flexor tendon management, 36-41. *See also*
   Tendon healing
   early controlled mobilization, 39-41, 40f
   general considerations, 36-38
   immobilization, 38
   passive motion, 39
Fluidotherapy, 199
Fractures, 191-223. *See also specific fracture
   type*
   basic principles, 191
   carpal fractures, 203-207
      hamate, 206
      lunate, 204-206, 205f
      schaphoid, 203-204
      triquetrum, 204
   distal radioulnar joint dislocation, 201-203
   distal ulna fractures, 201
   metacarpal fractures, 207-211, 207f, 208f,
      209f
      thumb, 210-211
   multiple fractures, 222-223, 222f
   pain management, 151
   phalangeal fractures, 211-221
      distal/intra-articular, 211-214, 212f, 213f
      middle/extra-articular, 214-217, 214f,
         216f, 217f
      middle/volar plate involvement, 217-
         220, 218f, 219f
      proximal, 220-221
   surgical management guidelines, 193-194
   therapeutic management guidelines, 194-
      195
   wound healing, 191-193, 192t
   wrist fractures, 195-201, 194f, 195f
Functional position splint, 175, 178f
Functional tests, 56

Group therapy, and pain management, 148-
   149, 149f
Guillotine-type injury. *See* Replantation
Gunshot wounds, 222-223

Hand therapy, history, 138
Hand/upper extremity functional unit, 160-161
Heat applications, 11, 12f-13f
Hypopathia, 151

Immobilization. *See specific anatomical area*; Splinting
Industrial hand injuries, 137-145
   case studies, 141-143
   history of hand therapy, 138
   physical capacity evaluation, 139-141
   work therapy, 138-139
Infection, and arthroplasty, 131-132
Inflammatory phase, of wound healing, 3-5
   management of, 5
Instrument tips, and sensory testing, 52, 53f
Internuncial pool theory, 71
Interphalangeal joint injuries
   distal level, 35-36
   proximal level, 33-34
Intrinsic healing, tendon, 22f, 23-24

Jobst garments, 100
Jobst jet air splint, 100
Joint contracture, 6
Joint jack splint, 179, 180f

Keinbock's disease, 204, 206-207

Letter identification, and sensory re-education, 60-61, 61f
Ligamentous anatomy, 163-164
Localization testing, 56
Localization training, and sensory re-education, 59
LMB active extension splint, 217
LMB wirefoam PIP extension splints, 104

Mallet finger, 212f
Materials, splinting, 168-169. *See also* Splinting
Matev distraction device, 214f, 215
Metacarpal fractures, 207-211, 207f, 208-209f
   and scar formation, 2-3
   thumb, 210-211
Metacarpophalangeal joint arthroplasty. *See* Arthroplasty

Metacarpophalangeal joint flexion/extension splint, 180-181, 182f
Minnesota Multiphasic Personality Inventory, 156
Minnesota Rate of Manipulation Test, 141
Motor function tasks, and sensory re-education, 62, 63f
Multiple fractures, 222-223, 222f
Muscle test, in replantation therapy, 101
Muscular anatomy, 162-163

Naloxone, 148
Neuromas, pain management, 151-152, 152f, 153f
Niebauer prosthesis, 120f
Nutrient pathways, of synovial tendon, 20f
Nutrition, and would healing, 5

Opiates, and pain management, 148
Opponens splint, 173-174, 177f
Optacon, 48-49
Oxygenation, and would healing, 5

Pain management, 147-156
   acutely injured hand, 149-150
   capsulotomies, 150
   carpal tunnel syndrome, 152, 154
   De Quervain's syndrome, 154-155, 155f
   early mobilization, 150
   endogenous opiates, 148
   fractures, 151
   group setting, 148-149, 149f
   neuromas, 151-152, 152f, 153f
   pain transmission theories, 147
   peripheral nerves, 151
   psychological aspects, 148
   reflex sympathetic dystrophy, 155-156
   tenolysis, 150-151
Pain transmission theories, 147
Paratenon, 19
Passive motion, controlled, and flexor tendon management, 39
Pattern theory (1927), 50-51
Peripheral nerve injury, 151
Phagocytosis, and wound healing, 4-5
Phalangeal fractures, 211-221
   distal/intra-articular, 211-214, 212f, 213f
      hand therapy, 214
   middle/extra-articular, 214-217, 214f, 216f, 217f
      hand therapy, 216-217

Phalangeal fractures (*continued*)
  middle/volar plate involvement, 217-220, 218f, 219f
    hand therapy, 219-220
  proximal, 220-221
    complications, 221
    hand therapy, 220-221
Phalens test, 154
Physical capacity evaluation, 139-141
Pressure testing, 56
Procaine, and reflex sympathetic dystrophy, 78
Prosthetic fracture, 131
Proximal interphalangeal flexion/extension splint, 104, 181-182, 184f-185f
Proximal interphalangeal joint arthroplasy. *See* Arthroplasty
Psychological aspects of pain perception, 148
Pulse Galvanic Muscle Stimullator, 197
Pulsed electromagnetic fields, 206
Purdue Pegboard, 141
Puzzles, and sensory re-education, 60-62, 61f, 62f

Radioulnar joint dislocation, distal, 201-203
  delayed complications, 202
  hand therapy, 202-203
Raynaud's phenomenon. *See also* Vasomotor disabilities
  anatomy, 72-73
  clinical manifestations, 73
  etiology, 70-71
  evaluation of, 73-74
  management, 82-85
    drug management, 85
    evaluation, 82-83
    long-term techniques, 83
    patient education, 84-85
    short-term techniques, 83
    surgical management, 85
    temperature biofeedback, 83-84
  nomenclature problems, 70
Reflex sympathetic dystrophy. *See also* Vaso-motor disabilities
  anatomy, 72-73
  etiology, 70-71
  management, 76-80
    baseline measurement, 76
    conservative management, 77
    pain, 155-156
    procaine management, 78
    splinting, 80
    steroid management, 78

  sympathectomy blocks, 78-79
  sympathetic management, 79
  temperature biofeedback, 79
nomenclature problems, 69-70
personality manifestation, 75-76
stages, 74-75
theories on, 71-72
Remodelling phase, of wound healing, 6-8
Renfrew ridge, 48
Replantation, 91-134
  case studies, 106-111, 112-113
  early ADL intervention, 99-100
  early post-operative management, 95
  early therapy phase, 96-97
  late phase evaluation and treatment, 100-105, 102f, 103f
  long-term problems, 113-115
  mobilization value, 98-99
  surgical considerations, 91-93
  technique, 93-94
  vocational psycho-social aspects, 105-106
  wound healing, 95-96
  wound management, 97-98
Retrograde milking massage, 197-198
Ridge test, 48
Rolando fracture, 210

Safe position splint, 174-178
Scar formation, 2-3
  and replantation therapy, 101-102
Scar tissue remodelling, 8-11, 9f
  the art, 10-11
  the science, 8-10
Schultz prosthesis, 121f
Semmes-Weinstein monofilament, 154
  test, 46-47
Sensation, defined, 45
Sensibility, defined, 45
Sensiometer, 48
Sensory recovery, in replantation therapy, 105-115
Sensory re-education, 57-64. *See also* Sensory testing
  activity selection, 63
  and functional sensation improvement, 58
  long term effects, 64
  rationale for, 58
  result asessment, 63-64
  methods of, 59-62
    discrimination training, 59
    games and puzzles, 60-62, 61f, 62f
    localization training, 59
    motor function tasks, 62, 63f

shape discrimination, 59-60
texture discrimination, 59-60, 60f, 61f
prerequisites for, 59
Sensory testing, 45-64
categories, 54t
historical perspective, 46-51, 47t
sensory re-education, 57-64. *See also* Sensory re-education
test interpretation, 57
test selection, 54-57
functional tests, 56
localization, 56
pressure, 56
static and dynamic spatial discrimination, 56
sudomotor, 57
touch, 54
vibration, 56
variables, 51-54
Shape discrimination, and sensory re-education, 59-60
Site selection, and sensory testing, 52
Smith's fracture, 195-201, 194f
Spasticity reduction splint, 176
Spatial discrimination testing, 56
Specificity theory (1895), 50
Splinting, 159-187. *See also specific anatomical area*
biomechanical principles, 167-168
forces, 168
levers, 167
pressure, 168
three point pressure system, 168
dual obliquity principles, 165
fabrication principles, 170-173
dynamic components, 172
patient education, 172-173
pattern design and material selection, 170-171
straps and closures, 172
working with material, 171-172
flexion creases, anatomy, 164-165, 164f
goals and purposes, 165-166
hand arches, anatomy, 161-162, 162f
hand/upper extremity functional unit, 160-161
ligamentous anatomy, 162-163
materials, 168-169
closures, 169
equipment, 169
list of, 183-184
types, 168-169
muscular anatomy, 163-164
osseous anatomy, 161

and reflex sympathetic dystrophy, 80
and replantation therapy
early intervention, 99-100
late phase, 102-104, 102f, 103f
supply list, 185-187
task analysis approach, 169-170
types of splints
dynamic, 166-167, 179-183
static, 166, 173-179
Stack splint, 212f
Static splinting, 166. *See also* Splinting
custom designed, 173-178
commercially made, 178-179
Steffe prosthesis, 121f
Steroids, and reflex sympathetic dystrophy, 78
Stress
in replantation therapy, 104
and scar tissue remodelling, 8-10
Sudomotor testing, 56-57
Surgical considerations, in replantation therapy, 91-93
technique, 93-94
Surgical management
fractures, 193-194
Raynaud's phenomenon, 85
Sympathetic management, and reflex sympathetic dystrophy, 79
blocks, 78-79
Synovial diffusion, and tendon healing, 20-21
Synovial sheath, and tendon healing, 25-27, 26f
Swan-neck deformity, 128-129
Swanson prosthesis, 120f

Tactile gnosis, 56
Temperature biofeedback
and reflex sympathetic dystrophy therapy, 77-79
and sensory testing, 51-52
and Raynaud's phenomenon, 83-84
Tendon healing, 18-41
extensor tendon management, 27-36. *See also* Extensor tendon management
flexor and extensor differences, 25-27, 26f
flexor tendon management, 36-41. *See also* Flexor tendon management
intrinsic vs. extrinsic healing, 22-24, 22f
phases of, 24-25
synovial diffusion, 20-21, 21f
vascular perfusion, 18-20, 19f, 20f
Tenolysis, 150-151
Test bias, in sensory testing, 53-54

Texture discrimination, and sensory re-education, 59-60, 60f, 61f
Theory of Head (1905), 50
Thumb fracture, 210-211
  complications, 211
  hand therapy, 211
Tissue healing, scars and, 2-3
Touch testing, 54
Transcutaneous nerve stimulation (TENS), 77
Trauma, and adhesion formation, 23
Two-Point Discrimination (2PD) test, 46

Ulna fractures, distal, 201

Valpar Simulated Assembly Work Sample, 139
Valpar Small Tools Mechanical Work Sample, 141
Valpar Upper Extremity Range-of-Motion Work Sample, 139
Vascular perfusion, and tendon healing, 18-20, 19f, 20f
Vascular reactions, and wound healing, 3
Vasomotor disabilities, 69-86. *See also* Raynaud's phenomenon; Reflex sympathetic dystrophy
  anatomy, 72-73

case presentation, 80-82
  etiology, 70-71
Vibration testing, 56
Vitamin deficiencies, 5
Vocational counseling, and replantation therapy, 105-106
Von Frey hairs, 46

Whirlpool treatments, in replantation therapy, 97-98
Work therapy, 138-139
Wound healing
  fracture, 191-193, 192t
  in replantation therapy, 95-96
  stages, 3-8, 3t
    fibroplasia phase, 5-6
    inflammatory phase, 5-6
    remodelling phase, 7-8
Wrist cock up splint, 175-176, 179f
Wrist flexion/extension splint, 179-180, 181f
Wrist fractures, 195-201, 194f, 195f
  early medical management, 195-197
  hand therapy, 197-201
    following cast immobilization, 198-201
    following closed reduction, 197-198
    post-fracture complications, 201

Zones of the hand, 21f